Totally
Buf

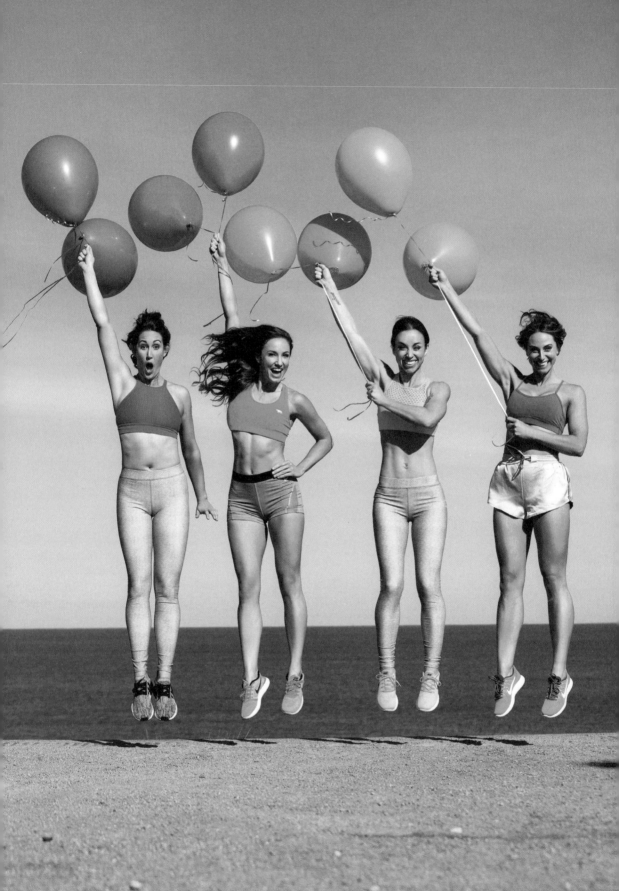

Your **6-WEEK GUIDE** to becoming BEAUTIFUL, UNSTOPPABLE + *fearless*

Totally Buf

LIBBY BABET & the *Buf Girls*

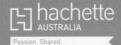
hachette
AUSTRALIA

Passion. Shared.

This book is dedicated to all girls around the world - the young and the wise.

Published in Australia and New Zealand in 2017
by Hachette Australia
(an imprint of Hachette Australia Pty Limited)
Level 17, 207 Kent Street, Sydney NSW 2000
www.hachette.com.au

10 9 8 7 6 5 4 3 2 1

National Library of Australia
Cataloguing-in-Publication data:

Babet, Libby, author.

Totally BUF : your 6 week guide to becoming beautiful, unstoppable and fearless / written by Libby Babet ; contributors: Cassey Miller ; Alicia Beveridge ; Sian Johnson .

9780733639364 (paperback)

Subjects: Women–Nutrition.
Physical fitness for women.
Physical fitness–Popular works.
Health–Popular works.

Other Creators/Contributors:
Miller, Cassey, contributor.
Beveridge, Alicia, contributor.
Johnson, Sian, contributor.

Internal design and layout by Liz Seymour, Seymour Design
Cover design by Neverland Studio
Images on cover, inside front cover and pages 4, 12–13, 16, 24–25,
    32, 40–41, 44, 54–55, 70–71 and 86–87 by Jody Pachniuk
Food photography and images on pages 5, 6, 7, 8, 94 and 95 by
    Steve Brown Photography
All other images courtesy of Next Realm Pty Ltd
Food styling by Bernie Smithies
Home economy by Kay Wijaya
Home economy assistants Helena and Vikki Moursellas
Colour reproduction by Splitting Image
Printed in China by Toppan Leefung Printing Limited

CONTENTS

INTRODUCTION

WHY WE WROTE THIS BOOK

Welcome to TOTALLY BUF, a six-week program designed to help you fall in love with living an active lifestyle, shift the way you think about your health and fitness, and build the kind of confidence and positive energy that comes from being part of an incredible community of like-minded women.

We believe getting healthy shouldn't be about focusing on weight loss, comparison and self-judgement but about leading an adventurous and fulfilling life. You need a strong, healthy body to be able to chase your goals, so concentrating on getting healthy for the right reasons, and finding joy in fitness, will help you create consistency and open up a world of possibility.

We're on a mission to put you on the path to helping you become the very best version of yourself, *and* set an incredible example for other women while you're at it. It's about letting go of stress, finding the fun in fitness and embracing real wholefoods that nourish your body. It's about finding your unique spirit and embracing the spirits of others. Perfect isn't all that interesting, but passionate, real and supportive sure is.

So often women tell us they find exercise hard and nutrition confusing, but this doesn't have to be the case at all. Simplicity is the key. As far as exercise is concerned, walking is more than enough, but group training, or connecting with an online fitness community, can make you feel part of something bigger, so that's a great next step. And when it comes to eating, simple wholefoods prepared with the best of

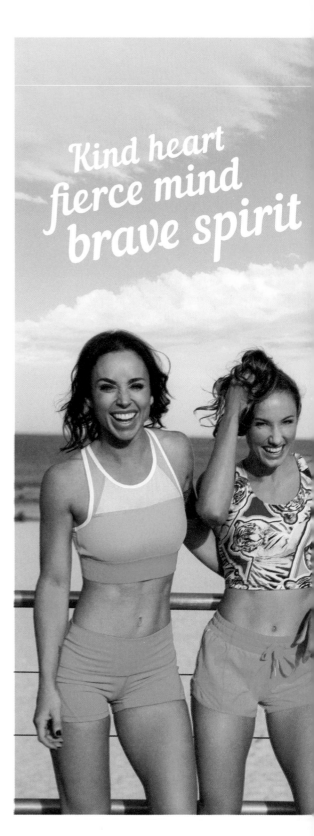

Kind heart
fierce mind
brave spirit

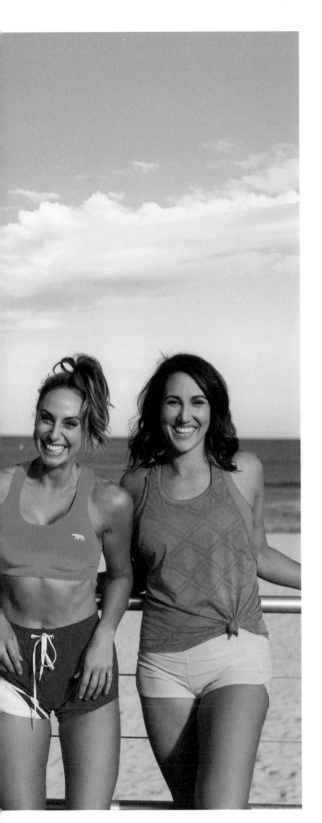

intentions are all you need. Processed food-like products drain your energy, and complicated 'foodie food' can be intimidating, but simple wholefoods make you feel lighter and happier.

The best things in life are simple. Healthy living should fit in with your life seamlessly, and feeling comfortable in your own skin is a positive side-effect of living a happy, balanced lifestyle.

BUF STANDS FOR BEAUTIFUL, UNSTOPPABLE AND FEARLESS.
This is exactly how we want to help you feel.

Being a BUF girl is about friendship and community. It's about healthy bodies and healthy minds. It's about inspiring, supporting and celebrating each other as the beautiful women we all are.

It's a shift *away* from dieting and battling against your own self-judgement and a shift *towards* eating well and moving often, because of how it makes you feel: happy, healthy, balanced, alert, calm, centred, strong, powerful, beautiful, unstoppable and fearless.

This book is designed to help you find your groove, create a balanced but flexible life you love, and embrace the wonderful body you've been gifted with. It's about approaching health the way you'd want a daughter or friend to approach it, from a place of excitement, balance, love, curiosity and understanding.

Bring on all that
girl power!

HOW TO USE THIS BOOK

The good news is, this book is not a diet book. You don't have to be super-motivated and organised to get incredible results from it. All you have to do is read one chapter a week, for six weeks. That's it.

Even if you don't make any of the recipes (although you should, they're incredible!), take any of the fitness actions or follow any of the meal plans, so long as you read each chapter as the weeks go by, changes will start to happen. Why? Because we've packed this book full of things you just can't un-learn once you've read them – things which will change the way you think about food and simple movement forever.

Each week you'll set one (B)eautiful intention, focus on taking just one (U)nstoppable nutrition action and complete one movement goal. We'll also help you create your (F)earless mindset with one thought-provoking task that will help get your head in the game, if you want to go a little deeper.

Every week has a meal plan, but you really don't have to use them. We've included these just for those people who love having a guide to reference and specific meals to create. If you need more flexibility, that's okay. Just adjust your regular dietary choices around the theme of the week.

For the vegetarian/vegans out there, we've provided swaps and suggestions for you in all recipes containing animal products.

It's totally fine to start with very small changes, and you might even feel you need to stick with one chapter for a few weeks before moving on, to totally nail it. That's cool.

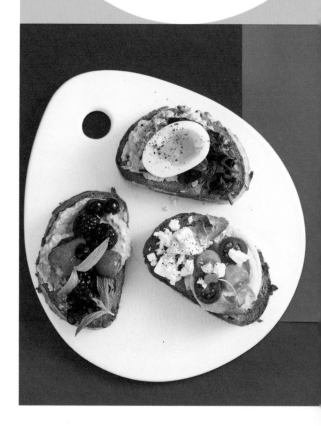

LIFE IS BETTER WHEN YOU'RE LAUGHING

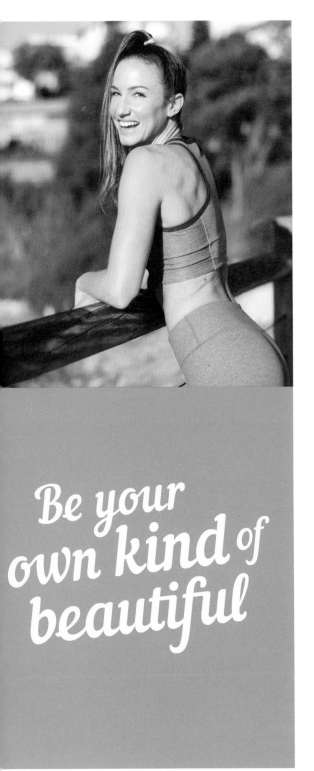

Be your own kind of beautiful

DON'T TRY TO BE PERFECT

This program is going to involve a little hard work, and there will definitely be challenges to overcome, particularly when you hit Curb Cravings week, but we guarantee that if you stick to the plan you will feel amazing and totally BUF by the end!

In accordance with the BUF Girls' spirit, 'sticking to the plan' doesn't mean you should try to be perfect – not at all. If you slip up with your nutrition, or just feel like a treat, that's fine. In fact, that's life. ☺

Don't feel guilty about it; just find your way back to the path at your very next meal or snack, and keep moving forward.

TRACKING YOUR PROGRESS

This process is all about learning to embrace your body, but it can still be nice to track your progress and celebrate when the healthy changes you're making start to show up with shifts in your body.

If you do have a goal then you need to know if you've achieved it, or how much progress you've made, and for that you need a starting point. Even if your only goal is to feel more energetic, it can be interesting and useful to see what changes happen to your body along the way.

Here's how we suggest you measure your progress ...

Take your measurements
(and put away the scales)

We recommend taking your measurements before you start and try to avoid the scales altogether, or at the very least only weigh yourself once at the start of the program and once at the end. This is because weight can be so misleading. For example, if you're weighing yourself every day you might find you gain weight at certain times of the month, or your weight loss plateaus for a

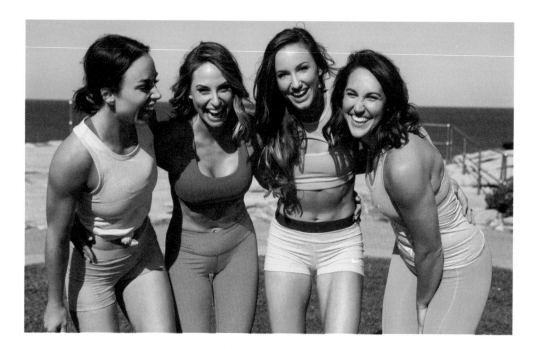

week as your body adjusts and you start to build a little lean muscle, all of which is normal but can be really demotivating if you're measuring your worth and progress by a number on a scale.

Chances are you will see significant changes in your measurements over the course of six weeks, so we recommend taking them at the beginning, halfway through and at the end. All you need is a measuring tape and you're good to go. Head to bufgirls.com/goals to learn how to take your measurements.

Before and after photos
Another quick and easy way to track your progress is to take some before and after photos. These are just for you - we're not asking you to share them. They can be a great reference point and powerful proof of your progress.

Start a food journal
This isn't necessary, but it is helpful for some people to track what they're eating and how each meal is making them feel. It's a great way to become mindful around what you're eating, and it can also be interesting to look back and see how you've progressed and changed your eating patterns over the course of the program. If you need a template, head to bufgirls.com/food-journal to download one.

IT'S OKAY TO BE A LITTLE NERVOUS!
Everything new is a little bit scary at first, but don't worry, you've got this! Courage isn't the absence of fear, it's moving forward in the face of fear.

If you need some extra support, rope a friend into doing this program with you, or join our community online at bufgirls.com where you can interact with other women getting totally BUF. We'll meet you there and you can ask any questions you might have, or voice any concerns. And to help you get an idea of who we are, here are our stories.

I'm the BUF Girls' founder and mission creator, tireless team supporter, megawatt energy generator, nutrition nerd, athlete maker, short shorts wearer, attempted surfer, multi-business starter and this book's author.

Libby

complete surprise of all my doctors, I stopped taking blood pressure medication and haven't looked back since. I'm not saying that's possible for everyone in my situation, but it happened for me and was a big wake-up call that how I treated my body and what I put in my mouth really mattered.

I believe I was put on this planet to help people feel good about themselves and live life to the full. Health and fitness has proven to be the most effective way for me to do that, because movement just makes people feel better!

The problem is, a lot of people are too scared to start a fitness program or turned off by a narrow image of what fitness is, and that's such a shame because fitness gives you the capability, the mental focus and the energy to get out there and make the most of your life.

I'm all about making fitness fun, exciting and interesting. I want to break down the barriers to getting started, draw people in and create strong communities around fitness where people feel loved, connected and like they belong.

I know what it feels like to struggle with confidence and health issues. In my early 20s I was diagnosed with chronic hypertension – my blood pressure was consistently more than double safe levels. Doctors had no idea what caused it, but told me I'd be on heavy medication for the rest of my life, which would harm my liver and make it difficult to have kids. It also gave me terrible skin, destroyed my confidence and created anxiety because I was at risk of suffering a stroke.

That wasn't good enough for me, so I decided to take control and started researching how I might be able to improve things, even just a little bit, through the right kind of fitness and nutrition. Within a few years of working closely with a number of specialists, to the

I was a journalist at the time, but this pushed me to become a personal trainer because the more I learned, the more passionate I became about sharing that knowledge. BUF Girls solved my own problem really. I'd gone through this huge life change and wanted to get back into exercise but the only options were super hard core, or way too serious. I could choose from getting a 'bikini body', training for a marathon, or weight lifting. It was either that or yoga and pilates, which are great, but I wanted something higher energy, and something that connected me to a community.

I was searching for something fun and uplifting. An experience that made me want to get up and go, then go back again the next day! So I created the 'entertrainment' experience. It all started with me, a few sets of dumbbells, a themed 'Beyonce Booty Circuit' and one brave client showing up solo. We had the best time ever, she spread the word and the next day there were two, the next month 20, by summer I was training more than 50 girls every morning.

Instead of making fitness a chore and nutrition a judgement, we were just having a blast, sharing information and creating principles we loved living our lives by, rather than following rules and stressing about our bodies.

Meeting Leash, Cass and Sian set my fate. The four of us coming together was really the start of the BUF Girls global movement and we've become sisters on a mission ever since!

I'm the butt-kicker, hike lover, tattoo addict, meditator, travel fiend, friendship fanatic, anxiety fighting, mascara fan girl, with impressive speed burpee skills.

Alicia
(Leash)

Fitness has always been part of my life in some way. At school I competed at state level in a range of athletics and the minute I was old enough to join a gym and jump into a few aerobics classes, I did. Being surrounded by others who loved fitness fuelled my passion for exercise, but I didn't think of it as a career option.

I spent years working in fashion at big magazines such as *Cosmopolitan*, but the industry didn't quite align with my personal values, so it was back to the drawing board! One day I saw an ad for a personal trainer's course, which was the first time it registered as an option for me. I applied straight away and the rest happened organically, as if it had always been written in the stars. Within weeks I was doing work experience with the fresh new kid on the block in Bondi Beach, Bottoms Up Fitness (now known as BUF Girls), and the rest is history.

Every challenge in my life has contributed to my resilience and tough spirit, but what I've been through has also brought out a really sensitive side that allows me to spot when others are feeling disconnected and reach out to help them feel welcomed and part of something.

When I was eight my father passed away from cancer and my mum struggled during this hard time. I spent time in foster care for a number of years, which meant I had to grow up pretty quickly and often felt displaced. This meant I floated between short-term stays with other families, never feeling I truly belonged. I became very good at searching for and establishing connections others may take for granted. Not having a solid family structure meant I had to work at finding love and being accepted, so creating those connections became a skill.

Even as an adult I suffer from anxiety and separation issues as a result of what I went through as a child, and my adult life has been a process of figuring all that out. Fitness has always been an important outlet for my stress and anxiety, a brief respite when I'm completely in the moment and focused on physical expression, just breathing and moving, rather than in my head, rehashing the past or worrying about the future.

I'm on a constant journey in terms of self-development and discovery, as despite having things mostly together as an adult, the challenges I faced when I was young still affect my day-to-day life. As we all know, life isn't always peachy, but suffering, anxiety and feeling alone are nothing to be ashamed of, and BUF Girls is about addressing all the parts of you that are holding you back from living your best life.

Creating a health movement based on connection, strength, empowerment, fun, laughter and courage has really helped me to become more open and honest about my own struggles, and has brought an incredible sense of freedom and contentedness.

Being a BUF Girl means being part of a family that celebrates, empowers, supports and uplifts everyone in it. It's about being the best you, not just for yourself but for those around you who'll benefit from your confidence and clarity. It's about holding the health of your mind and body in high regard, knowing success follows self-care and being real, perfectly imperfect, inclusive and warm.

I'm the good vibes maker, curves creator, white sneaker and red wine lover, fun chaser, celeb trainer, sisterhood believer, loyalty lover, fashionista, booty toner, and BUF's resident smiling assassin.

Cassey

I love helping women to achieve their best in all areas of life, by lifting them up with positive words, encouraging movement every day and providing knowledge so they feel empowered to make the right decisions when it comes to healthy living.

I do all of this with a sprinkle of fun and playfulness because that is how I believe life should be. Creating good vibes everywhere I go!

I've spent much of my adult life in the corporate world working in amazing jobs, including being promotions manager for Red Bull, flying around the world as an airline hostess with Emirates and selling luxury champagne for Moet-Hennessy! However, I found the corporate world insanely stressful and didn't feel I ever really fitted in with the busy office and harsh sales environment.

I'd never been an athlete, just an average kid at school sports who always gave it a go. My mum was the one who got me into exercise when I was about 18. She used to drag my teenage butt to aqua aerobics and the gym. It took her a while to convince me that it was doing any good but eventually I stopped reading magazines while cruising on the bike waiting for her to finish and got serious.

I started training with the BUF Girls as a client back in 2012 and their approach to nutrition and training was the only program that actually changed my body shape significantly, while also taking the pressure off and helping me fall in love with fitness.

All of a sudden, I wanted to work out because it made me feel happy, strong and healthy, not because I felt I had to. I loved the energy, passion, knowledge and authenticity that all the trainers had and knew I needed to be part of this crew. I completed my training course, quit my full-time job, said goodbye to my company car and phone and said hello to my new life as a trainer. I've never looked back!

One thing I love to do is prove to women how fitness can instantly connect them to a fun community no matter where they are in the world. I love to travel, try new fitness experiences and capture it all on video to show people back home where the most welcoming places to train are.

Life has not always been smooth sailing for me and the moment I fell even more in love with the BUF Girls community was when I separated from my husband. The love, support and new connections that flooded in when I was in a time of need meant the absolute world to me and I am so grateful to be part of such a caring crew of amazing, like-minded women. Surrounded by love on all sides, our communities both online and in person flooded me with good vibes until I felt safe, loved, worthy and centred again.

I've learned how to slow down and really look at my thought patterns, listen to my body and be as gentle and forgiving with myself as I would be with others.

Being a BUF Girl is not just about doing a workout or eating a healthy meal, it's about being part of a caring, accepting, supportive girl squad, creating new friendships, achieving balance, focusing on happy, healthy bodies and minds, and of course generating plenty of good vibes every day!

I'm the booty shaker, self-love preacher, tree climber, podcast devourer, non-stop giggler, puppy dog obsesser, camping rookie, triple-threat diva, and daggy fashionista.

Sian

My lifelong love has been dancing! I started young and became totally hooked, loving the fact that it combined fitness, social time, a creative outlet and my passion all in one! It was through my dancing that I developed a love for musical theatre and I just knew this was something I had to pursue.

After years of intense training I finally hit the big time and kicked my legs as high as I could, eight shows a week in the Australian tour of *A Chorus Line*. It was a total dream come true and a memory I'll cherish forever.

As much as I loved the performing industry, the dancing, singing, costumes, bright lights and let's be honest, the accolades ... there were also some very challenging aspects. Image was everything. I was constantly faced with the question of whether my body was right for the role. Was I tall enough, thin enough or even pretty enough to make it up on that stage?

Although these judgements grated on my confidence, they also helped me find a strength and resilience and discover value in the incredible things my body could do (like a triple pirouette into a leap) rather than the way it looked. I decided not to let my worth be defined by my image, and as I transitioned out of performing and into the world of fitness, I naturally gravitated towards training women to share that message.

At first I was shocked that so many of the incredibly beautiful, wonderful and talented ladies I was training felt they weren't all of

these things because their body didn't meet society's 'ideal' image. I realised everything I had overcome as a performer, I could now share to help make a difference.

At the beginning, I was disheartened because it seemed every time I instilled one positive thought, at least five negative images would flock into these girls' minds through channels such as social media and advertising. I felt that until we could change the dialogue around body image and fitness and what it truly meant to be 'healthy', nothing would shift. I couldn't do this on my own so I set off on a mission to find my tribe!

I was looking for a team of strong and inspiring women who trained not for the perfect body, but for a better lifestyle; who built other women up rather than exploiting their imperfections; and who embraced the joy in life by celebrating every moment together as a community. That's when I found BUF Girls and I knew immediately I'd found my place.

Being a BUF Girl is about doing everything for the love of it. Training because you love your body and want to keep it fit and healthy, eating because you love the way nourishing your body makes you feel, and building a strong mindset of self-love that allows you to be courageous and fearless each and every day!

Surrounding yourself with a super like-minded girl squad can make you feel unstoppable and remind you how beautiful you are, inside and out.

I love, Love, LOVE my body and I want every girl out there to feel the same way. The minute we can let go of that internal battle over self-worth, the sooner we can understand that it's our actions and the value we add to the lives of those around us that defines us.

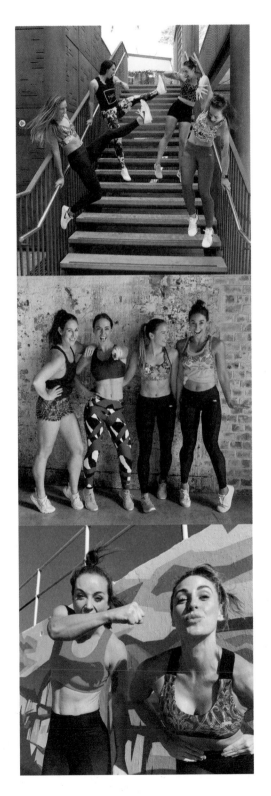

HOW OUR RECIPES WORK: HEALTHY MEALS AS EASY AS 1, 2, 3

Calories, portions, nutrition labels, complex recipes, healthy ingredients, organic or not, processed or fresh, paleo, low-carb, ketogenic, macros ... *gaaah*! Sometimes, choosing the right way to eat and preparing healthy meals is all too hard, which is exactly why we created the BUF healthy meal model. This three-step approach to creating your meals is all you need to know to start drastically improving your health. And the good news is, it works for every body type.

All you have to do is make sure that every meal or snack includes these three elements:

(B)eautiful, nutrient-packed plant foods - vegetables and/or fruits

(U)nstoppable energy foods - quality proteins and/or slow-release carbohydrates

(F)earless fats and flavours that create happy hormones and healthy appetites

That's it!

We'll get to fancier things a bit later in the book. For now, just worry about *what* you're putting in, not how much. Trust your appetite, eat slowly, and create your meals with our 1, 2, 3 guide.

When you turn to our recipes at the back of the book, you'll see that we've split your ingredients into B, U and F categories, dividing them into vegetables/fruits, proteins/carbs, and fats/flavours, so you always know you're getting a balanced meal.

Here are some examples of what a 'BUF' meal might include:

BREAKFAST – (b)eautiful chopped broccolini, kale, mushrooms and spinach leaves, tossed in a pan with (u)nstoppable energy from a few beaten eggs, and some (f)earless fats and flavours from coconut oil and fresh avocado (see Sautéed Greens Bowl recipe, page 128).

LUNCH – (b)eautiful green salad leaves, chopped tomatoes, pumpkin, rocket, capsicum and cucumber with (u)nstoppable energy from grilled chicken and quinoa, and (f)earless fats and flavours from tahini, avocado and olive oil (see Rainbow Abundance Bowl recipe, page 166).

AFTERNOON SNACK – (b)eautiful slices of green apple, (u)nstoppable energy from a tablespoon of almond butter spread on top of the slices, which also contains plenty of (f)earless fats, and you can add extra flavour with a sprinkle of cinnamon on top

DINNER – (b)eautiful leafy greens, (u)nstoppable energy from half a cup of cooked brown rice, (f)earless fats from smoked salmon (this has protein too, but also lots of healthy omega 3 fats), topped with avocado and a delicious, healthy dressing (see Brown Rice Poke Bowl recipe, page 140)

LEARN THE LINGO – WHAT THE HECK ARE THESE?

Macronutrients These are energy sources that the body needs relatively large amounts of. The three macronutrients required by the human body are carbohydrates, fats and proteins.

Carbohydrates These are the sugars, starches and fibres found in fruits, grains, vegetables and milk products.

Fats The fats derived from food provide your body with essential fatty acids that fuel a lot of vital functions in your body, support brain and nerve health and help you to absorb a lot of critical fat-soluble vitamins from your food.

Proteins These are the important building blocks of bones, muscles, cartilage, skin, hormones and blood. Proteins are found in animal products like meat, seafood, eggs and dairy foods, but also in beans, quinoa, buckwheat and a few other grains, along with nuts and seeds, spirulina and other algae, chia, hemp and soy.

Wholefoods When we refer to wholefoods, we mean food that has been processed or refined as little as possible and is free from artificial substances.

STOCK UP THE FRIDGE

Before you start this program it's a good idea to clear out your cupboards and stock the fridge with fresh ingredients that will fuel your week. The following list should cover all the different sorts of foods you'll need for success.

Vegetables All the green and colourful veggies you can find, like broccoli, cauliflower, beans, asparagus, capsicum, beetroot – anything goes. When it comes to starchy vegetables like potatoes, enjoy them but don't go overboard. Our favourites are pumpkin and sweet potato.

Salad All the salad ingredients your heart desires: lettuce, sprouts, tomato, avocado, cucumber, baby spinach.

Fruit Fresh, in-season fruit, ideally organic if you'll be eating the skin but if not just wash it all well and you're good to go. BUF Girls' tip: berries, apples, stone fruits and citrus are the lowest-sugar fruits.

Juices No fruit juice, except for maybe a squeeze of lemon in warm water in the mornings, but if you have a juicer or a favourite café with delicious options, feel free to drink fresh vegetable juices, ideally based on greens like spinach, celery, cucumber, maybe a little carrot, beetroot or half a green apple to give it taste. You'll learn all about why we're ditching fruit juices in Week Two!

Meat and Fish Plenty of lean (ideally organic or at least hormone-free) protein sources, plus oily fish like salmon and sardines, and small white fish. Try not to rely on tuna, as it can contain a lot of heavy metals so can be bad for long-term health, especially if you're trying to conceive. A small amount is okay, though.

Eggs Free-range eggs – up to two per day gets the okay from the powers that be these days! Hard-boiled eggs are great as snacks.

Nuts Unsalted nuts and seeds, ideally pre-soaked/activated (this makes them easier to digest), but otherwise raw or dry-roasted.

Dairy Dairy is cool if you can tolerate it, but always go for full-fat, plain organic yoghurts and milks, used in moderation. You'll see why as we get into Week Four. Take note how you feel after consuming dairy, as some people have intolerances that can affect digestion, skin or mood. Alternative options are sheep's and goat's milk, yoghurt and cheeses, and coconut and almond milk products.

Carbohydrates Sweet potato, corn, beans, rice, quinoa, seeds/nuts, fruit, rice and buckwheat are all great sources of fuel.

Snacks Concentrate on wholefood snack sources, like nuts, seeds, chia, fruit, vegetable sticks and hummus. Ditch packaged biscuits, muesli bars and other processed goods.

Protein powder We'll delve into this in detail in your first week, but we do use protein powder in a few of our recipes, and teach you how to pick a good one. If you want to be sure, though, we've created our own, hand in hand with some of the most incredible foodies in the land. It's vegan and it's delicious! Grab yours at bufgirls.com/protein-powder.

Treats If there are a few treats you really love, check the back of the pack and look for minimal ingredients, make sure you recognise those ingredients, and look for less than 5 g of sugar per 100 g and zero trans fats. Doesn't fit the bill? Don't buy it!

Ready to get stuck into your program?

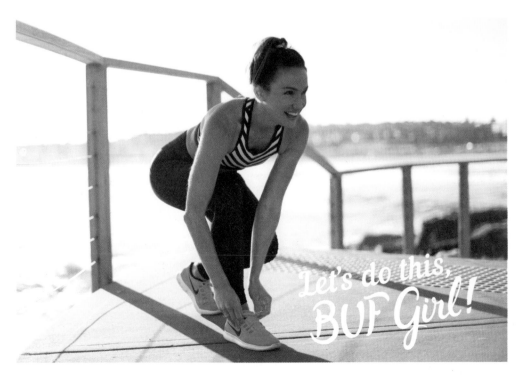

Let's do this, BUF Girl!

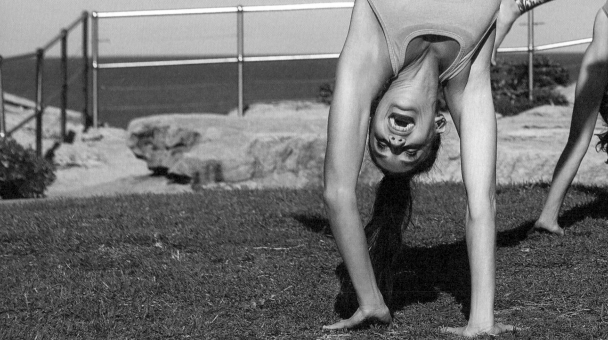

Boost your Energy

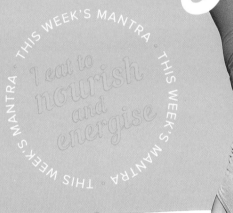

THIS WEEK'S MANTRA · THIS WEEK'S MANTRA · THIS WEEK'S MANTRA · THIS WEEK'S MANTRA ·

I eat to *nourish* and *energise*

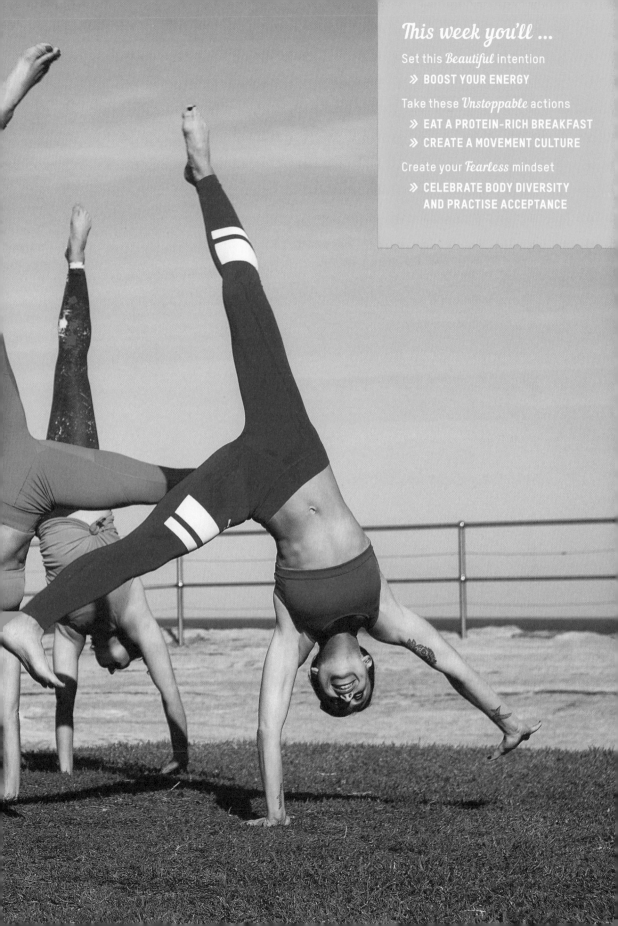

This week you'll ...

Set this *Beautiful* intention
» **BOOST YOUR ENERGY**

Take these *Unstoppable* actions
» **EAT A PROTEIN-RICH BREAKFAST**
» **CREATE A MOVEMENT CULTURE**

Create your *Fearless* mindset
» **CELEBRATE BODY DIVERSITY
AND PRACTISE ACCEPTANCE**

» Boost your energy

Welcome to Week One of your **Totally BUF** adventure! This week is all about filling your body with energy.

Now, the first reaction we get from women who read that statement is usually, 'Boost energy? But I want to change my body! How many calories should I be eating? What *exactly* should I be doing every day?'

We hear you ... we've all been there! But there's a good reason we do things differently at BUF Girls. You see, anyone can follow a short-term plan and get fitter and leaner for a little while, but most of the time that initial motivation fades and before long you're right back where you started. The goal of this particular program is to help you create and maintain an incredible, healthy, happy, connected and seriously fun life that you are committed to, long-term.

But to create any big shift, you need to generate some serious momentum, and to create momentum you need a whole lot of energy! This is why we focus on boosting your energy first.

» Eat a protein-rich breakfast

Ditch starchy, low-nutrient breakfasts like packaged cereal, toast, muffins and pastries and replace them with good-quality proteins, vegetables and fats.

The reason we're focusing on this particular action right off the mark is that it can make a HUGE difference to how you feel and the way your body uses energy. In fact, we may go so far as to say that taking this action alone could change your life.

Here are five reasons for making this one simple change to your first meal of the day:

1   You'll be burning (rather than storing) energy from your very first meal of the day.

2   Overall fat-burning metabolism increases.

3   Your energy levels are more likely to be consistent, without peaks and crashes, so you can say goodbye to those desperate 10 am coffee runs and devastating 3 pm slumps.

4   You're likely to feel more focused and driven, with increased stamina.

5   You'll be packing in more nutrition, right from the outset.

DON'T GET STUCK ON THE REFINED CARBOHYDRATE ROLLERCOASTER!

Rollercoasters are fun at first, but riding one all day long would drain your energy pretty quickly, right? That's exactly what happens when you start your day with carbs. Your blood sugars spike quickly and you get a hit of energy, then they crash just as fast and you're ravenous or feeling moody and low. If you set this pattern at the start of the day, you're stuck riding the rollercoaster all day long, constantly looking for little pick-me-ups.

BUF Girls are definitely not paleo preachers, but it's fair to say that, genetically, humans haven't evolved too much since cavewoman times, so it makes sense to eat in a similar manner to how our ancestors ate – and those boxes of sugary cereal sure don't grow on trees!

WHAT'S SO WRONG WITH CEREAL ANYWAY?

The majority of breakfast cereals are far too high in sugar and salt, as well as being heavily processed and laced with preservatives, additives and colours. Unless you're just eating plain oats or unroasted, very low-sugar muesli with no extra oils or dried fruit added, most cereal is:

1   high in energy density (calories)
2   high in refined carbohydrates (which quickly break down to sugar in your body)
3   low in nutrients (leaving you low on energy)
4   high in chemicals, preservatives, oils or salts (which can put stress on your body)
5   kinda unsatisfying (they don't fill you up for long)

Check your cereal box label and you'll often see sugar (or a substitute like honey, agave, rice syrup, or anything ending in 'ose') high

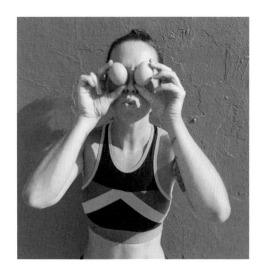

up on the ingredients list, which is not what you ideally want to be putting into your body when you break your fast.

For serious cereal lovers who want to reintroduce some cereal after this week of protein-based breakfast eating, you might like to make your own muesli. Toss together a few cups of plain rolled oats, a big handful of shredded coconut, a few tablespoons of chia seeds, a handful of mixed nuts and a tablespoon or two of your favourite fibre-packed dried fruit (we love goji berries). Store in a jar and you've got a bulk stash of goodness ready for those too-rushed-to-cook-or-think mornings.

WHAT ABOUT TOAST?

There's nothing wrong with a good-quality slice of sourdough, rye or grainy toast as a bed for your eggs, avocado or greens. However, bread on its own is not a very nutritious food, so if your breakfast consists of a few pieces of toast slathered with spreads, it's worth asking the question, 'What am I missing out on because I'm filling up on this? Is this going to boost my energy with lots of body-loving nutrients, sustaining protein and hormone-loving fats, or is it just a filler?'

SO, WHAT TO EAT FOR BREAKFAST THIS WEEK?

Approach breakfast as you would lunch or dinner. That means filling your plate with all the good stuff …

Start with a clean protein source like eggs, lean organic meat, smoked fish, natural yoghurt, a homemade vegan protein shake, tempeh, or brown rice combined with beans (this combo creates a complete protein!). Next, add a small amount of healthy fat like avocado, nuts or seeds, soaked chia, a drizzle of olive oil, a little tahini or some organic butter. Finally, include some extra fibre, ideally from vegetables or a small serve of whole fruit.

Be fearless of eating healthy fat. Fats fill you up quickly and satisfy you for longer, which means you end up snacking less. They also nourish your hormones, help with mental clarity, stabilise your moods and can definitely help you reach your body goals. Refined sugars, added salts, and processed and unhealthy fats like the ones you find in deep-fried foods and many packaged foods, are the real enemy. Often 'diet' options are low in fat but high in sugar and additives, confusing your appetite and wreaking havoc on your digestion.

WHAT DOES ALL OF THIS HAVE TO DO WITH BOOSTING MY ENERGY?

Carbohydrates, especially the refined or 'simple' types, enter the bloodstream quickly, especially first thing in the morning when your body's been fasting for a number of hours. Because these simple carbs are easily broken down into sugar once inside your body, with little or no fibre to slow down the rush, this gives you a quick burst of pleasure and alertness as blood sugar levels rise quickly, followed by an equally fast drop in energy and mood when your body responds to the sugar dump by releasing a huge amount of insulin to 'mop it all up'.

The adrenal glands (your stress regulators) also respond to this drop in blood sugar levels by activating your 'fight or flight' response and pumping out the stress hormones adrenaline and cortisol to try and make you feel a little better. However, the adrenals are not designed to work all the time – they are the emergency 'energy boosters' of the body. In time, they can become depleted and your fatigue may become chronic.

When you experience the symptoms of low blood sugar, like irritability, fatigue,

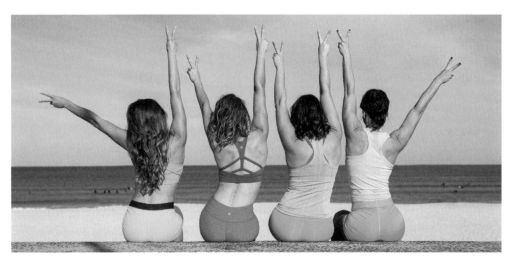

hunger or a 'fuzzy head', you feel like you desperately need a quick carbohydrate hit to pick you up again, which kicks off another spin on the rollercoaster, and so the ride continues.

Take a stand! It's up to you to break the cycle by choosing foods that provide slow-release energy for your body to use throughout the day. And it all starts with breakfast.

SCORING BONUS BRAINPOWER

Neurotransmitters are chemical molecules in your brain that play a role in the way you behave, learn, feel, perform, think and even sleep.

Complete proteins not only contain a stress-busting amino acid called tyrosine, they also encourage the release of neurotransmitters such as dopamine, a potent motivation booster, serotonin, which keeps your mood upbeat, and acetylcholine, which increases memory and focus, supports physical activity and combats anxiety.

This means that instead of feeling lethargic, moody and stressed out, eating protein at breakfast can actually help fire you up for a really successful day of work or play.

Pretty cool, right!

WINNING THE VENDING MACHINE WARS

So, you've eaten a protein-dense breakfast and balanced your appetite hormones, you're feeling all fired up and you're humming along nicely, but we know you're wondering ... will the office vending machine still be calling your name by 3 pm?

It's common to feel hungry or low in energy mid-afternoon, as a dip in your stress and

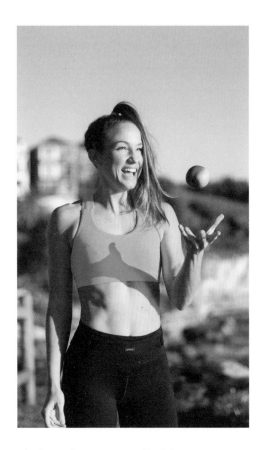

alertness hormone, cortisol, happens around this time of day. What your body really needs now is more protein and nutrients to perk it up, not a chocolate bar that's 50 per cent sugar, 25 per cent chemicals, 15 per cent colours and fake flavours and 10 per cent goodness-knows-what.

By sneaking in another mini protein hit at this time of day, you'll increase your metabolic rate and also boost your energy and focus for the afternoon, all while reducing cravings for those vending machine tempters.

Pairing your protein choice with something slightly sweet can be a good idea, so you're still satisfied and feel you've had a 'treat', without resorting to those brightly packaged food imposters behind the shiny glass.

WHAT ELSE CAN YOU DO TO BOOST ENERGY?

Drink more water!

As little as 2 per cent dehydration can affect your energy levels, leaving you feeling drained and fatigued. You don't necessarily have to follow the 'eight glasses a day' rule, but you do want to drink enough water to keep your body well hydrated, so make sure you keep a bottle on your desk, or take a walk to refill your glass every 60–90 minutes – the walk will give you a little hit of incidental exercise, too!

And the next time you feel that 3 o'clock crash coming on, have a glass of water or a mug of herbal tea before you reach for the snack jar.

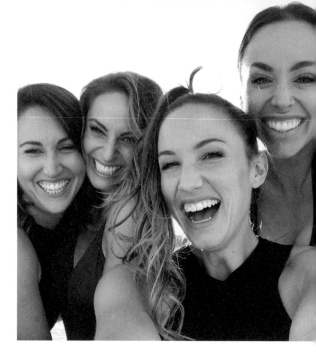

Get more sleep

If you're not winning in the sleep stakes, try these tricks to hit reset.

1 Prioritise sleep when you can, even if you have other things to do. We promise it will make you so much more productive tomorrow!

2 Be consistent – sleeping short all week and trying to 'catch up' on weekends just doesn't work.

3 Cut down on caffeine – a cup or two in the morning isn't going to hurt, but caffeine is a stimulant that disrupts sleep, so having a pick-me-up mid-afternoon can really affect the quality of your zzz's.

4 Don't drink alcohol too close to bedtime – it disrupts the way your body flows from one sleep stage to the next. This means if you're sipping on wine too close to bedtime, you might wake with a start in the middle of the night and struggle to doze off again.

5 Ditch the screens at least an hour before your head hits the pillow – the blue light from your TV, laptop or phone screen stimulates your brain and puts you on the no-sleep train. An e-reader with a low light is fine, or read an old-fashioned book, go for a walk or just spend time with the people you love.

6 Create a pre-bed routine – just like kids, adults respond well to a solid evening structure that helps them nod off. An hour before bedtime, have a shower or bath, read a book, meditate … whatever takes you from stimulated to sleepy.

7 Drink a drowsy tea – valerian or chamomile will help you bust stress and chill out.

8 Try a new kind of alarm clock – if you generally get up when it's still dark, try picking up a dawn simulator. These incredible alarm clocks slowly wake you up with a half-hour of 'sunrise' that totally feels like the real thing.

9 Grab a magnesium supplement, or even better a magnesium oil to rub on your stomach and under your feet before bed, to help you de-stress and sleep soundly.

ALL ABOUT PROTEIN SHAKES

One of the questions we always get asked during boost-your-energy week is, 'If the focus is on having protein for breakfast this week, can I just use a protein shake?' The answer is pretty simple. If you can meet your daily protein needs through wholefoods, that's the best way to do it.

However, what protein powders are great for is convenience. If you need a quick breakfast on the go, an energy-replenishing meal you can eat on your way from the gym to work, or something

really great, most of them are packed with artificial flavours, synthetic vitamins, sugar, artificial sweeteners or low-quality ingredients.

All you really want to see in the mix is the plain protein, plus maybe a few natural ingredients to create flavour, like vanilla, dried coconut or cacao. If the blend contains a natural sweetener like stevia or xylitol, that's okay too. You definitely want to avoid thickeners and fillers, which will make it much harder for your body to digest any of the good stuff.

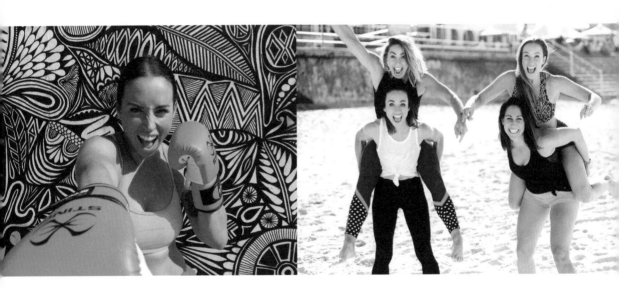

to keep in your bag in case you need a snack and don't want to hit the vending machine, having a serve of good-quality protein on hand is such a winner. Protein powders are also amazing for use in making protein-rich snacks, adding to your baking, boosting protein intake for vegetarians and vegans, or recovering from really intense exercise, particularly weight training.

How to choose a protein powder

There are SO many protein powders on the market, and while some of them are

We believe if you're consuming protein powders regularly, vegan options are the best, as they're usually easier to digest and less likely to have side effects if you overdo it. Go for a pea, rice or hemp-based protein.

The best options for animal-product-based proteins are whey, casein or cricket flour (yep, you read that right: crickets are an excellent and environmentally friendly protein source!). Steer clear of soy-based proteins unless suggested by your health pro, as they can affect your hormones.

» Create a movement culture

So many women come to us feeling exhausted after years of taking the 'all or nothing' approach to their health and fitness.

We've all been in that place at one point, working out every day or not at all, trying the latest fad diet only to regain that weight the following month, signing up for a gym membership and only walking in the door once.

In our cumulative 25+ years of training women, we've found the cause of yo-yo'ing fitness levels is most definitely *not* a lack of willpower, it's a lack of meaning. In other words, you know what to do, and you know how to do it, but you're just not sure you want to actually do it, and you're not in the habit of doing it.

Here's how to fix that in 3 steps:

1   Replace the word 'exercise' with the word 'movement' and make moving a habit you practise all day long, as often as possible, not just when you have time to hit the gym. Walk between meetings, take the stairs, park a few blocks away from your destination and walk the extra distance. Roll out of bed and do 10 push-ups, 20 squats and 30 star jumps to wake yourself up; go for a walk around the block every 2 hours at work; play active games with your kids after work; stretch in front of the television instead of eating in front of it. **Create a movement culture that becomes part of how you live your life.**

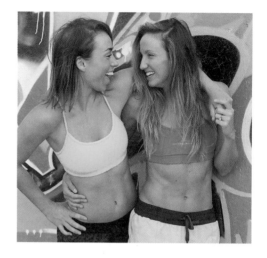

2   Link your movement culture to your core values. Is it family you value? Move because your kids love it and it sets a great example, or walk with your partner because it gives you tech-free, meaningful time in each other's presence. Is it a successful career you value most? Move more and eat well because the healthiest employees are up to three times more effective than the least healthy! Is it helping others that brings you joy? Learn everything you can about health and fitness, then live and breathe it so you inspire others. **Linking your core values in life with healthy habits makes all the difference.**

3   Understand that habits are incredibly powerful once they're in motion, but getting there will take effort. Did your mum need to remind you to brush your teeth every day when you were a kid? Ours sure did. But we brush every morning and night now, without thinking about it. **We are what we repeatedly do.**

THIS WEEK'S (F)EARLESS MINDSET » Celebrate body diversity & practise acceptance

When starting out on a physical journey it's important not to neglect your mental training, because it really is true that if you get your mind in shape, the body will follow.

Just like fitness improvements, getting to a place where you respect and accept your body takes time, repetition and consistent effort. Every single woman has thoughts like, 'I can't do this', or, 'I'll never have a body like that', but there are some easy ways to redirect those thoughts and get your mind working for you rather than against you.

To create lasting change, it's important to shake up the story you're telling yourself about all the things you 'should' be and take a moment to accept and appreciate where you're at right now. That doesn't mean you can't still want to create some serious change, it just means you stop putting yourself down and comparing yourself to others.

Let's start with a little gratitude practice and give a voice to all the awesome things that make you you! Write down the following:

The most (b)eautiful part of my body is

....

My body can do this really incredible thing that makes me feel (u)nstoppable. It is

....

The personality trait that makes me so (f)earlessly unique is

....

Need some girl power to get you started? Here are a few of our answers!

Alicia The most beautiful part of my body is ... my waist. My hips and bust are on the larger size, so my small waist makes me feel womanly and curvy.

Cassey My body can do this really incredible thing that makes me feel (u)nstoppable. It is ... sprinting! I would not call myself a 'runner', as I'm not a fan of long-distance runs, BUT get me on a treadmill for a 250 m sprint and you can see me at top speeds of 20 km per hour!

Sian The personality trait that makes me so (f)earlessly unique is ... my passion! It's like a great big fire in my belly that drives me to constantly challenge myself and those around me to be the best we can be!

Libby Celebrating and being grateful for all the great things about being you is a very empowered place to start your journey from.

> BEING HAPPY DOESN'T MEAN EVERYTHING IS PERFECT, IT MEANS YOU'RE WILLING TO LOOK BEYOND THE IMPERFECTIONS

TOP TIPS 'n' TAKEAWAYS

» This week, eat to nourish and energise your body.

» Start your day with a protein-packed breakfast to feel focused and energised.

» Include a little healthy fat and fibre to keep your appetite hormones happy and to feel fuller for longer.

» Create a movement culture by looking for as many opportunities for movement throughout your day as you can.

» Focus on wholefoods for your other meals and snacks.

» Drink lots of fresh water (herbal tea is great too!).

» Create a pre-bed routine and wake up fresh.

» Practise a healthy body image. Focusing on acceptance and habits that create little moments of happiness is much less exhausting and more energising than chasing perfection.

WEEK ONE

MEAL PLAN

	Breakfast	*Lunch*	*Dinner*
MONDAY	Baked Eggs in Mushrooms PAGE 101	Bacon and Broccoli Salad PAGE 130	Ricotta and Mushroom Zucchetti PAGE 214
TUESDAY	Chia Pudding with Almonds and Goji Berries PAGE 106	Raw Broccoli Salad with Curry Cashew Dressing PAGE 168	Brinner Frittata PAGE 184
WEDNESDAY	Naked Breakfast Bowl PAGE 124	Chicken, Haloumi and Beetroot Salad PAGE 146	Oven-baked Fish and Chips PAGE 206
THURSDAY	Nutty Granola PAGE 116	Triple C Patties with Asian Slaw PAGE 174	Raw Pad Thai PAGE 212
FRIDAY	Sautéed Greens Bowl PAGE 128	Grated Salad with Tahini Dressing PAGE 134	Chicken-Stuffed Sweet Potatoes PAGE 190

Snack options

» PROTEIN-PACKED SUPER SMOOTHIE (PAGE 245)

» PRO YOGHURT (PAGE 234)

» APPLE WITH NUT BUTTER (PAGE 242)

» BLEND 'EM EGGS (PAGE 235)

Curb Cravings

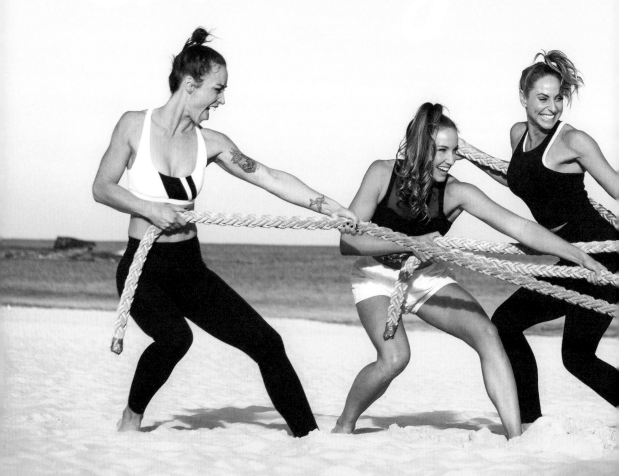

This week you'll ...

Set this *Beautiful* intention
» **CURB CRAVINGS**

Take these *Unstoppable* actions
» **BE A SUGAR-FREE SISTA!**
» **TRY WORKOUT SNACKING**

Create your *Fearless* mindset
» **EAT MINDFULLY TO ENJOY YOUR FOOD MORE AND RESPECT YOUR BODY'S APPETITE CUES**

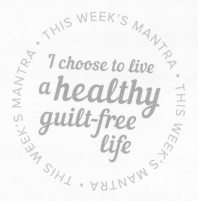

THIS WEEK'S MANTRA • THIS WEEK'S MANTRA • THIS WEEK'S MANTRA • THIS WEEK'S MANTRA •

I choose to live
a healthy
guilt-free
life

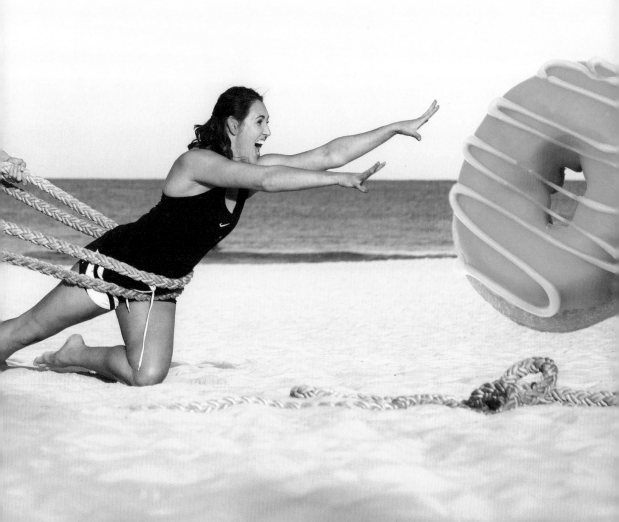

» *Curb your cravings*

Let's get one thing straight. Cravings are not a sign of weakness, they're not your fault, and more than that, sometimes it would be a crime not to give in to them. After all, life is for living, and who could possibly enjoy living without the odd serve of chocolate, glass of wine or handmade loaf of bread? Not us!

So many women we work with beat themselves up for giving in to cravings, often using one treat as a reason to give up on healthy eating for the rest of the day and feeling a deep sense of guilt when they do 'give in'.

But food is not the enemy and we are all hard-wired to enjoy it, so you're not alone in wanting to reach for a few squares of chocolate straight after dinner, even though you've just eaten a hearty meal. Everyone's been there, and it's okay from time to time.

However, when it goes beyond the odd treat and you start to develop a habit of overeating, or struggle to stop at one serve of your favourite sweet food, it becomes difficult to move on in your health journey.

The good news is, curbing your cravings is not just about cutting things out. Eating enough of the right foods, eating regularly, understanding why you crave certain foods at certain times, having alternative options handy, eating mindfully and continually up-skilling your nutrition knowledge will help put a stop to the cycle of addiction.

USE PRINCIPLES, NOT RULES, TO SLAY EVERY DAY

Curbing cravings and achieving your healthiest body shape is not about creating a strong set of rules to stick to, because you know as well as we do that as soon as you set a rule, you just want to break it! To combat cravings, all you need to do is learn to create a set of principles to live your healthy life by.

When it comes to weight loss and living your healthiest life, the important thing to

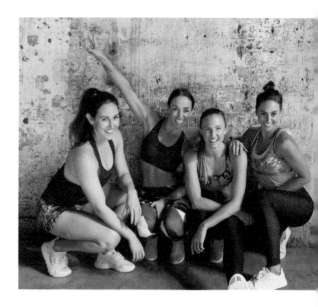

note is that it's the nutritional value of your food that matters, not the amount of energy, or calories, it contains. Even someone with no knowledge of nutrition could probably tell you that eating 1200 calories of deep-fried potato chips is going to have a very different outcome for your body than eating 1200 calories of wild salmon and steamed vegetables.

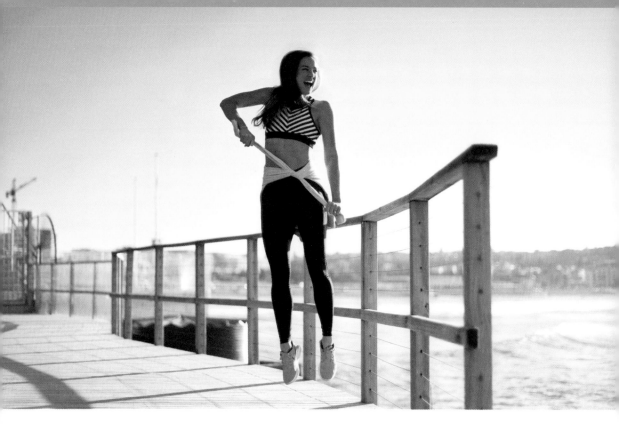

A great principle to use instead of the calorie rule might be, 'I choose to eat real, unprocessed food that's as close to its natural state as possible whenever I can.' Or, 'I am a healthy person and aim for a balanced meal of protein, healthy fats and fibre each time I sit down to eat.' If you tend to overeat, a good principle might be, 'I always eat slowly and mindfully, enjoying my food and paying attention to hunger cues.'

These principles are flexible and simple to stick to, because they make sense. Plus, you can literally use them as little mantras before meal times to remind you of the healthy life you have created for yourself. They feel good, not restrictive!

SO WHEN SHOULD YOU START THINKING ABOUT CALORIES?

Your number one intention should be to establish a good base of consistently-healthy eating before worrying about the more intimate details of calorie input/ output and nutrient timing. Most women get better and longer-lasting results this way.

Once you've firmly established healthy eating habits, it can be interesting and sometimes helpful to be roughly aware of the calorie content of foods you eat regularly, so you know you're not overdoing it. Calorie counting is also helpful for athletes who need to get really specific about their food intake, and for pregnant and breastfeeding women who might need to bump up their energy needs.

But for most of us, if you manage your portion sizes and are mindful of putting quality foods into your body, you won't have to worry about counting calories.

An alternative might be to keep a food journal in which you record everything you eat and drink for seven days, plus what size portions, then review it at the end of the week. Take note of any habits you have that may be holding you back, or whether you need to up your vegetable intake, or water count, and so on. As mentioned on page 4 we have created a template that might be helpful for this, at bufgirls.com/ food-journal.

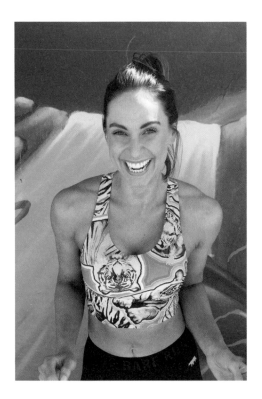

We don't stress about eating 'super clean', and we definitely have little treats when we crave them, but we choose the best-quality version of those treats and don't overdo it, always getting right back to nourishing our bodies at the very next meal or snack.

Interestingly, each of us remembers a time when we were younger and less educated about health when we *did* stick to calorie-counting diets and were a lot less in control of our body shapes than we are now, dealing with yo-yo'ing weight and moods. During those years we were eating significantly fewer calories than we are now, and almost half the amount of food, but a lot of it was packaged, low-fat or 'diet' convenience foods that were high in refined sugar, additives and preservatives.

Better bodies with more calories? Chalk up a big WIN for healthy food, and plenty of it.

QUALITY ALWAYS WINS

No matter what new fads hit the market, all our years of working with women have proved to us that it's the quality of your food and the balanced range of nutrients you're getting that really counts when it comes to feeling satiated and turning your body into an efficient energy-burning machine.

Curious about how many calories WE eat? All four of us compared our daily food intake while we were writing this section, and when we added up the calories we discovered that, over the course of a week, our individual calorie intake varied every single day – anywhere from roughly 1400 to 2400 calories per day, depending on how busy we were and what we had on.

There were also variations in routine every day – some days we ate three square meals, sometimes it was two meals and a few snacks, and on other days it was closer to six small meals spread out across the day.

We've all maintained our body shapes for years now, eating in this relaxed way, so there goes the idea you'll automatically put on more weight if you eat more calories, or don't eat the same amount at the same time every single day. The thing is, most of what we're eating is really nourishing food.

Ultimately, curbing your cravings for foods that aren't helpful, and maintaining a functional, efficient metabolism is often about adding more food, not taking food out. And isn't that a relief!

That said, this week we *are* going to take something out. We want you to experience what it's like to live for one whole week without refined sugar in your diet, so you can create a circuit-breaker in that cycle of addiction and enjoy the energy-boosting benefits that come with getting off the sugar rollercoaster.

» *Be a sugar-free sista*

Now that you're in the habit of eating protein and healthy fats for breakfast, your blood sugar levels will be more stable and you should be starting to feel a lot more energetic, so it's the perfect time to add another super-powerful nutrition habit to your list. Your nutrition focus for the next seven days is on cutting as much refined sugar as possible from your diet, while also cutting down a little on natural sugars, too.

The goal is to reset your palate, reduce cravings and break the addictive hold sugar can have on your body, to calm that sweet tooth, balance appetite hormones and give your digestion, liver and brain a fresh start.

What this means for you over the next seven days is:

1   No sweet drinks, including sports drinks and soft drinks, even the 'diet' kind, and no adding sugar (not even honey!) to your tea/coffee.

2   Reduce alcohol significantly. Stick to a maximum of one glass, and go for red wine, or clear spirits (vodka, gin, tequila) with soda water and a wedge of fresh lime or lemon.

3   No sugary desserts and zero visits to the vending machine, unless you find a packet of nuts hiding in there somewhere!

4   No processed snacks containing sugar or sugar alternatives.

5   Check nutrition labels and ditch foods (even 'health foods') containing more than 5–10 g of sugar per 100 g.

6   Limit sugary sauces (most tomato sauces, for example, contain almost 50 per cent sugar). Stick to the basics: mustard, apple cider vinegar, fresh lemon/lime juice, olive oil, hot chilli with no sugar added.

7   Ditch 'low-fat' products with hidden sugars: low-fat cheeses and flavoured yoghurts, fruit cups and ice-creams. Again, stick to options with 5–10 g sugar per 100 g.

8   Say goodbye to fruit juice and dried fruit. Limit fresh fruit intake to just 1–2 serves per day, ideally sticking to low-fructose fruits like berries, green apples and citrus.

9   No substituting for 'fake' sugars/ sweeteners, with the exception of stevia, xylitol or monk fruit, which are safe, plant-based sweeteners. Even then, use in moderation this week, as they can encourage sweet cravings.

10 Limit starchy foods that have the same effect as sugar on your body – things like white bread, crackers and white rice break down into sugar as soon as your body starts digesting them.

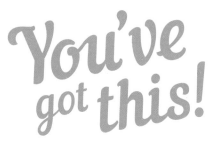
You've got this!

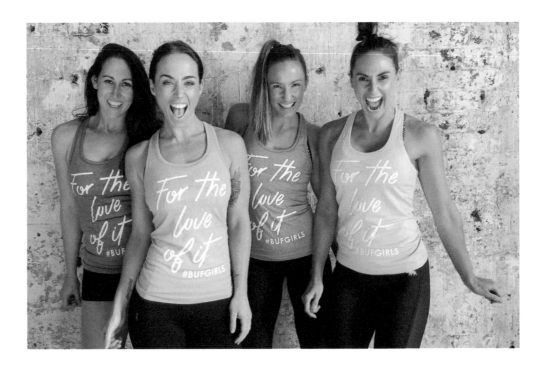

Signs you need some sugar-free time

If you answer 'yes' to any of the following, this week will be hugely beneficial for you:

- Do you get an energy slump in the afternoon?
- Do you feel like you 'need' something sweet after meals?
- Does your stomach get bloated after eating?
- Are you holding weight around the midsection?
- Do you often feel jittery and 'starving' between meals?
- Do you feel like you need to eat every few hours to keep your energy up?
- Are you craving coffee mid-morning and mid-afternoon?
- Do you find it hard to resist the office sweets jar?
- Are you anxious about cutting your favourite foods out this week?
- Do you consume certain foods, even if you're not hungry, because of cravings?
- Are your favourite foods sweet rather than savoury?
- When cutting out sugar for even one day, do you suffer from headaches, moodiness or low energy?
- Do you struggle to stop at just one sweet, baked good, biscuit or cracker?
- Are you a latte or cappuccino lover who shudders at the thought of drinking an unsweetened espresso or long black?

If you've answered 'yes' more than a few times, it's time to reset your palate!

You'll find after just seven days without sugar, your tastebuds will change significantly and a lot of the above symptoms disappear. Not only that, a simple apple will start to taste amazing, and you'll be surprised how sickly-sweet some of the things you used to love begin to taste.

WHY IS IT SO HARD TO SAY NO TO SUGAR?

Firstly, humans are biologically tuned to seek out sweet things. In nature, the only truly sweet foods are fruit and honey, which are seasonal and hard to find but also packed with important nutrients and vitamins, so your body is hard-wired to enjoy them.

So many of us also grow up emotionally and physically attached to sweet foods, from the moment we're given our first glass of orange juice as a child, or bribed to behave with a few jelly snakes. If you feel tangible fear at the thought of not being able to turn to something sweet when you're feeling low, tired or bored, or as a way to celebrate a victory or milestone, you're not alone. But if giving up your sweet treat 'reward' trigger means you may be rewarded with a clear mind, lean body, increased focus and more stable emotions, isn't it worth a go?

GIVE ME THE HARD FACTS! WHY SHOULD I EAT LESS SUGAR?

A lot of really healthy, natural foods are broken down into sugar in the body, including vegetables and fruits, complex carbohydrates and sometimes proteins, but that process happens slowly and gives your body time to use the energy as it's breaking it down. The issue with refined sugars and processed carbohydrates is that they provide a pretty extreme amount of energy that is rapidly delivered to the body, and anytime you've filled your body with more fuel than it needs, excess fat storage occurs. That's not so bad every now and again, but if you're consistently swallowing sugary treats, your body will consistently be storing fat and never burning it, which not only sabotages your body goals but can increase inflammation in your body and make you feel fatigued, which then encourages more cravings as you try to 'pick yourself back up'.

Here are a few other reasons kicking the sugar habit is worth doing:

- When you eat sugar and refined carbohydrates, the hormone insulin is released in high levels. Insulin is responsible for shuttling blood sugars into storage in your liver, muscles or, most often in the case of sweet foods, fat tissue. After insulin has mopped up all the blood sugar, there's often a delay in the time it takes for your body to stop releasing the hormone, which leads to a big dip in blood sugar levels, causing an immediate spike in appetite, encouraging you to eat more.

- When a post-sugar-intake 'crash' occurs, your body releases a rush of the stress hormone cortisol, which encourages your body to release stored sugar from the liver to stabilise blood sugars. That extra glucose meets the energy coming in from your next snack, and once again your body is in a state of stress, releasing more insulin to deal with the situation.

- The combination of readily accessible sugars coming in for your body to burn and the consistent over-production of insulin to deal with those sugars can prevent existing stored fat from being released and used up as energy, because your body literally can't burn fat when insulin is present and doing its job.

- If you consistently eat sugary foods, your hormonal balance and liver function can be compromised, resulting in outcomes like weight gain, allergies, immune system weakness, chronic fatigue syndrome and disease risk.

- Sugar can increase depression, anxiety and inability to focus.

- It can interfere with digestion, increase bloating and lead to the malabsorption of food and nutrients.
- Sugars can directly interfere with your brain's communication with leptin, the hormone that suppresses your appetite. So your likelihood of overeating and obsessively craving not-so-wholesome foods increases.
- High sugar intake has been linked to high levels of inflammation in the body, which can increase joint pain significantly.
- You'll age more quickly on a high-sugar diet, as it causes cell structures to harden and increases wrinkling.
- Refined sugar is incredibly addictive. Experts now compare it to tobacco and even cocaine in terms of its addictive and harmful properties.

Convinced you don't need that afternoon sugar hit yet?!

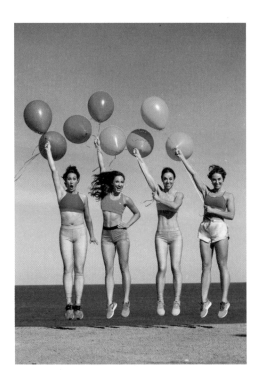

SO ... HOW MUCH SUGAR IS TOO MUCH SUGAR?

According to national guidelines, the following is what you need to know. (Note that daily sugar recommendations are based on 'free sugars', which include added sugars, those found in refined sugars and processed foods, but also natural sugars found in things like honey, agave and other syrups, as well as fruit juices and concentrates. (Not included are the sugars found in milk, vegetables and whole fruits.)

- Women should have no more than 6 teaspoons of free sugars per day. Men can have up to 9 teaspoons, and for children the general recommendation changes depending on their age but ranges between 3 and 7 teaspoons.
- Try to stick to foods with less than 5–10 g of sugar per 100 g (check the nutrition panel every time you purchase a new product).
- 1 teaspoon of sugar is roughly 4 grams, so that means your upper limit per day should be 25 g of free sugars.

To put this in perspective, one small can of soft drink typically has around 10 teaspoons of sugar (that's nearly double your daily dose!), sports drinks have 9–10 teaspoons, a small cup of fruit juice has at least 5-6 teaspoons, a tub of flavoured yoghurt can have up to 7 teaspoons, 1 slice of banana bread has around 11 teaspoons, and milk chocolate has 1 teaspoon per square (by comparison, dark chocolate containing around 85% cocoa only has 1 teaspoon per 3–4 squares).

WHAT CAN YOU SWAP THESE FOR?

When you're trying to give up your favourite foods, it's handy to have some substitutes ready. Try these direct swaps for the foods we listed above:

- Swap soft drink for mineral water – infuse it with some fruit for extra yumminess.
- Swap sports drinks for fresh water with a small squeeze of fresh orange, or a pack of hydrolyte if you're an endurance athlete and need to replace electrolytes.
- Swap fruit juice for a piece of real fruit, or a green vegetable juice (think spinach, celery, cucumber, kale, parsley, lemon).
- Swap fruit yoghurt for plain Greek yoghurt (or alternatives like coconut yoghurt, or sheep's milk yoghurt), with fresh berries and a few nuts or seeds stirred in.
- Swap banana bread for these simple cookies: mix 2 ripe bananas with 1 cup of oats, shape into biscuits, drizzle with coconut oil and bake for 15–20 minutes at 200°C.
- Swap milk chocolate for good-quality dark chocolate, or a warm mug of boiled water with a heaped teaspoon of unsweetened cacao or carob powder, sweetened with some coconut milk and a little stevia.

Note that sugar comes hidden under many other names, such as sucrose, glucose, high fructose corn syrup, maltose, dextrose, raw sugar, cane sugar, malt extract and molasses. Pretty much anything else ending in 'ose' is a sugar. Be careful of artificial sugars, too. Research now tells us that artificial sweeteners can be just as bad for our health as refined sugar, perhaps even worse, messing with our bodies' hunger signals, heart health and ability to process carbohydrates, so try not to just swap one for the other.

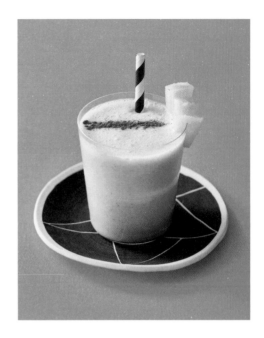

WHAT ABOUT ALCOHOL?

There's no getting around it, alcohol does contain sugar, and not only that, your body prioritises metabolising alcohol over everything else, which can affect the way you're able to digest and utilise other food while it's in your system. The good news is that a lot of the fructose is burned off in the fermentation process, so things like dry white and red wines, or clear spirits, are fairly low in sugar.

More important is to watch what you're mixing your alcohol with. Mixers are often loaded with sugar or chemical alternatives, soft drinks are obviously a sugar bomb, tonic water has the same amount of sugar as a can of coke, and mixing alcohol with highly sugared or very creamy liquids can lead to increased fat storage and poor digestion.

It's also worth noting that most cocktails contain some kind of sugar, syrup or fruit juice, so check with the bartender and put in an order for something a little more 'straight up'.

You don't have to give up the booze completely to be healthy, but sticking to just 1 or 2 glasses, 1 or 2 times per week, is a good guide.

ATTACK OF THE AFTER-DINNER MUNCHIES!

For most people, the evening meal rarely finishes when the dinner plates hit the sink. Even after a meal that leaves you full to the brim, chances are that as soon as you're done you'll be hunting for a 'finisher'.

Habit is the major cause of reaching for something sweet following a meal, and if eating dessert has been a tradition for you since as long as you can remember, chances are you'll never feel quite satisfied until you've had something sweet, despite how full you are, because your mind is looking to retrace old habits. Combine a strong sense of habit with the fact sweet treats also make you feel happy in the short-term by elevating the mood-boosting chemical serotonin, and you've got a pretty addictive little combination.

But don't despair, there are some strategies to help steer you away from the fridge once dinner is done.

One is to **set yourself an eating curfew**. If you usually have dinner at around 7 pm, give yourself a mental curfew of 7:30 pm and don't eat after that time. You can even make a sign that says 'Kitchen Closed', and when curfew hits, stick it on your fridge or pantry – a fun little reminder that, just like at your favourite café, when the kitchen's closed there are no orders being taken.

Just brushing and flossing your teeth can do the trick, or drinking a soothing digestive tea. Another strategy is to **go for a walk**, or use your favourite TV show as a time to do a few squats, sit-ups and push-ups at every ad break. Not only will this give you something to do that doesn't involve eating, it will also get you moving!

Guilt-free treats – try these on for size! If you are going to snack once your main meal is out of the way, at least do it right ...

- Melt some chocolate that's at least 80% cacao and dip fresh strawberries in it. Place on a lined tray in the fridge to set. Portion them up and enjoy a few each night.
- Pop some popcorn kernels on the stove using a little coconut oil, or organic butter, then sprinkle with cacao or cinnamon powder.
- Eat a spoonful of organic peanut or almond butter. Even better, scoop your spoonful into a small bowl and stir in the teeniest bit of melted coconut oil mixed with cacao or carob. (Warning, this is seriously addictive!)
- Eat fresh, organic mixed berries with a scoop of full-fat Greek yoghurt and a sprinkling of stevia powder.
- Have a scoop of cottage cheese with one finely chopped date mixed into it.
- Munch on a small handful of frozen grapes – red tastes best!
- Make a creamy, yummy chia seed pudding. Simply pop a tablespoon or two of chia seeds in a cup, cover with coconut milk, sprinkle with cinnamon and allow to set in the fridge for 10 minutes.
- Indulge in a few squares of low-sugar chocolate.
- Bake an apple. Just pop it in the oven for 10–15 minutes until soft. So yummy! For extra luxe, serve with a scoop of coconut yoghurt.

» Try workout snacking

Think of motivation as being like a fire. It won't get lit if you don't take some very important little actions first. Step one is to place twigs and paper in the hearth and set a match to them, then you have to add some bigger sticks and finally, when it's really going, a large log or two. Voila! You have your roaring fire.

If you had sat there waiting for the fire to appear out of nowhere, nothing would have happened. And if you'd put the big log on before the smaller sticks, it would have put out the flame.

This is often what happens when people set big fitness goals like, 'I want to lose 10 kilos' ... it's just too overwhelming. You have to start with the little actions (the small twigs that get the fire started) – short workouts, walks at lunch time, active play with your kids. By repeating these actions consistently you can turn them into big habits.

That's where workout snacking comes in!

Workout snacks are bite-sized bits of movement you can use to fire yourself up for a big day, to boost energy after lunch, to blast a little stress after a big day or just to make exercise manageable.

We love to swap afternoon snacks for workout snacks, because movement has been proven to boost energy more effectively and for longer than eating a sugary snack, and often moving your body will push away cravings, too.

Here are five workout snacks you can try next time the munchies hit, or when you need a little pep up:

1   A brisk walk around the block – the original and the best workout snack!

2   The 10-to-1 snack, where you choose two exercises and do 10 repetitions of each of them, then 9 of each, then 8, 7, 6, 5, 4, 3, 2, 1. You can keep it as simple as squats and push-ups, or get tricky with burpees and crunches, or try star jumps and high knee runs on the spot.

3   A 4-minute Tabata snack: pick an exercise, do it for 20 seconds with as much intensity as you can, take 10 seconds rest, repeat eight times through for a total 4-minute energy booster.

4   The skipping snack: just 10 minutes of fast-paced rope skipping can burn as many calories and improve your fitness as much as a 30-minute run.

5   The Primal Seven: do 10 repetitions of 6 of the 7 primal movement patterns to wake up your entire body! The patterns are: squat, lunge, hinge (i.e. bodyweight 1-leg deadlifts), push, pull, rotate (i.e. trunk twists).

Life has ups and downs, we call them **squats!**

» *Eat mindfully* (why not try living that way too?!)

These days we are so caught up in the rush, always 'on' thanks to technology and social media, that eating isn't the sacred rest time it used to be. The shift this creates in everything from your digestion to the amount you eat and the way your body uses the food is enough to have a serious impact on your health, waistline and mindset.

Casually introducing some mindful eating habits can make a huge difference. Here are a few ideas for you to try out this week:

Give your body time to catch up to your brain

Your body sends it's 'I'm full' signals to your brain about 20 minutes after eating, so speed-eating can mean you miss those important cues and end up overeating. Try putting your fork down between bites, chewing well (as many as 20 times for each bite) and swallowing before picking up the fork again. And really *taste* your food. See if you can pick out every flavour!

Ditch the distractions

Multi-tasking and eating is a recipe for disaster, because it makes it a lot harder for you to pay attention to hunger signals and encourages you to eat on auto-pilot.

Try creating these habits:

1 No eating in front of a screen, whether it's a TV, computer or Instagram feed.
2 Try not to eat in the car as you rush between commitments.
3 After dinner, go for a walk or have a stretch, rather than plonking on the couch straight away while you're still in 'eating mode'.

Pause before you snack A lot of people use the term 'emotional eating', but really that's just another form of eating without being mindful of your body's needs first. Stopping to check in with where your body is at – and if you're really hungry, or just bored, lonely, sad, procrastinating, distracted or low in energy – can be a powerful habit.

Try doing these things before your next snack:

1 Ask yourself, 'What are my emotional hunger triggers?' and pay attention to them next time you go to reach for a snack. Consider whether you are really hungry, or just hoping for a distraction.
2 Aim to leave 3–4 hours between each main meal of the day, and 12 hours between dinner and breakfast. Just having this simple structure in place gives you a guide as to when to eat and when to hold off.

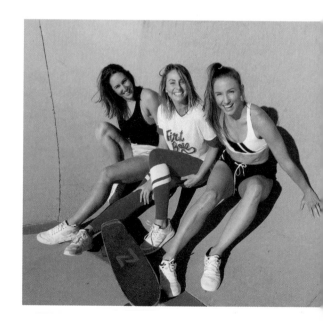

3   Use the 'drink before you dig in'
    rule. Make a big cup of tea (we love
    peppermint, chamomile, chai and
    lemon/ginger), or pour yourself a glass
    of water, and drink slowly before you
    decide whether or not to reach for a
    snack. Sometimes when you feel hungry
    you're actually just thirsty, or in need of
    something to do with your hands!

Feel like a changed woman!

WRITE YOUR MANTRA

Every time a negative thought pops into
your head this week, write it down, then flip
it and stick your new mantra somewhere
where you can find it easily next time you
need to reverse your thinking.

Here's how to do it: simply write down
the unhelpful thought, then switch it to
the exact opposite and write that down
too. For example, 'I'm so unfit' becomes
'I'm committed to getting just a little
bit fitter every day', 'I can't give up junk
food' becomes 'I choose to fill my body
with nutritious food', and 'I hate the gym'
becomes 'I love moving my body to fill it
with fresh energy'. Practise sitting quietly
for 60 seconds, breathing in deeply and
repeating your mantra on every out breath.

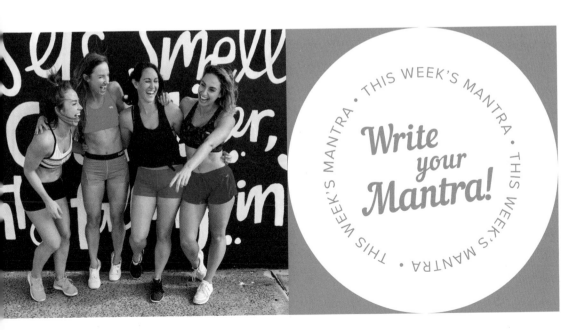

THIS WEEK'S MANTRA • THIS WEEK'S MANTRA • THIS WEEK'S MANTRA • THIS WEEK'S MANTRA

Write your Mantra!

TOP TIPS 'n' TAKEAWAYS

» This week is about choosing to live a healthy, guilt-free life.

» Eating too many simple carbohydrates, especially from refined sugars, encourages the body to store unhealthy amounts of fat, whereas slower-release carbohydrates are more likely to be used as energy and moved out of the body.

» Refined sugars can skyrocket your insulin levels, kick-starting an energy rollercoaster that will only end in more cravings.

» Before you sit down to a meal, ask yourself how nutritious it is and whether it fits the BUF healthy-eating model. It's okay to have treat meals sometimes, but most of the time your meals should contain the healthiest available ingredients that are as close to their natural state as possible.

» Learn how to create your own simple meals, desserts and sauces that don't have sneaky hidden sugars in them.

» The national Heart Foundation recommends a maximum of 6 teaspoons of free sugars per day for women and 9 for men. One teaspoon of sugar is roughly equal to 4 g – this is helpful when checking labels, as you just divide the total by 4 to get the approximate amount of teaspoons (e.g. 12 g sugar = about 3 teaspoons).

» Eat mindfully to enjoy your food more, and respect your body's appetite cues.

MEAL PLAN

	Breakfast	*Lunch*	*Dinner*
MONDAY	Appetite-balance Smoothie PAGE 100	Mixed Roast Veg with Chicken PAGE 154	Beef Satay Stir-fry PAGE 182
TUESDAY	Basic Omelette PAGE 102	Pumpkin and Broccolini Salad with Walnuts PAGE 164	Ginger and Garlic Fish Parcels PAGE 181
WEDNESDAY	Avocado and Feta Smash PAGE 100	Cauli-fried Rice with Chicken PAGE 142	San Choy Bao Balls PAGE 218
THURSDAY	Easy Peasy Protein Pancakes PAGE 109	Chickpea, Orange and Goat's Feta Salad PAGE 132	Roast Chicken with Carrot and Pumpkin Purée PAGE 216
FRIDAY	Vanilla Orange Overnight Proats PAGE 125	Homemade Sushi PAGE 138	Mexican Mince and Bean Bowl PAGE 198

Snack options

» AVOCADO AND CHICKPEA HUMMUS WITH VEGGIE STICKS (PAGE 243)
» ALMOND-FLOUR MUFFINS (PAGE 232)
» CAROB, BANANA AND MACADAMIA LOAF (PAGE 237)
» MUG OF TRIPLE C GOODNESS (PAGE 244)

I choose the **healthiest** *version of the food I'm* **craving**

WEEK THREE

Swap, don't Stop

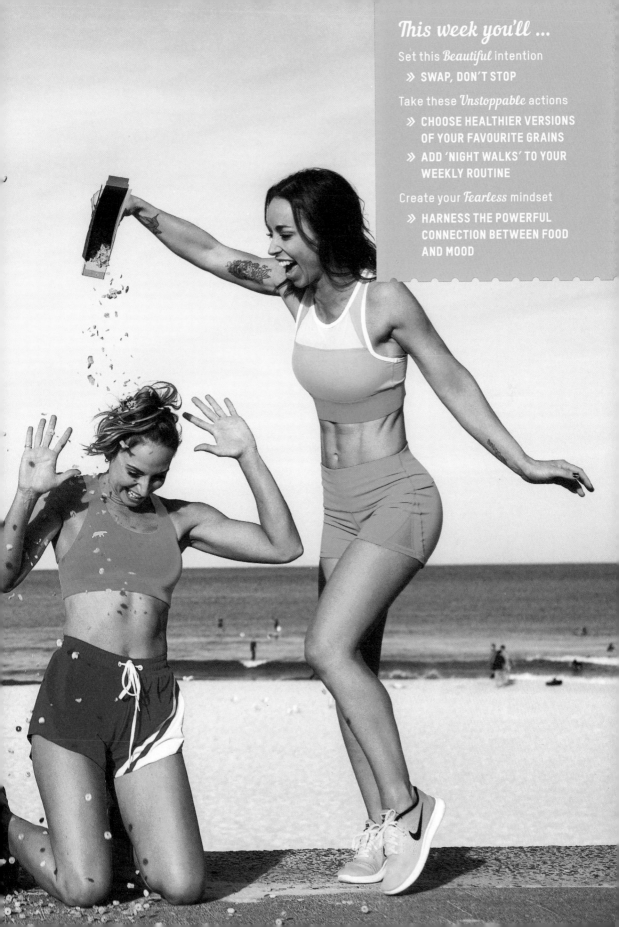

This week you'll ...

Set this *Beautiful* intention
» SWAP, DON'T STOP

Take these *Unstoppable* actions
» CHOOSE HEALTHIER VERSIONS
OF YOUR FAVOURITE GRAINS
» ADD 'NIGHT WALKS' TO YOUR
WEEKLY ROUTINE

Create your *Fearless* mindset
» HARNESS THE POWERFUL
CONNECTION BETWEEN FOOD
AND MOOD

» *Swap don't stop*

Week Three is the time to put your health-nerd hat on and figure out the science behind getting grains right, as well as experimenting with whether gluten-containing grains are right for you.

Consciously choosing to eat the healthiest available versions of your favourite foods, and making sure you're always asking yourself, 'How is this serving my body?' is a really great habit to get into.

Ask yourself this: if you were given a million-dollar racehorse tomorrow, would you feed it deep-fried, processed food with little to no nutrition, jack it up on caffeine all day so you can race it harder, fill its drinking trough with alcohol and sugar every night, and keep it up late staring at a screen? Sounds like a pretty great way to send your million bucks to an early grave! Not only that, treat a horse like that and it's pretty likely to end up skitty and anxious, stressed out, low in energy, with unpredictable moods.

So why do we treat our own priceless bodies this way? It's time to treat your body like the precious, wonderful gift that it is.

And the up-side? Choosing 'healthier' most of the time means you can choose 'anything goes' every now and again without any negative side effects.

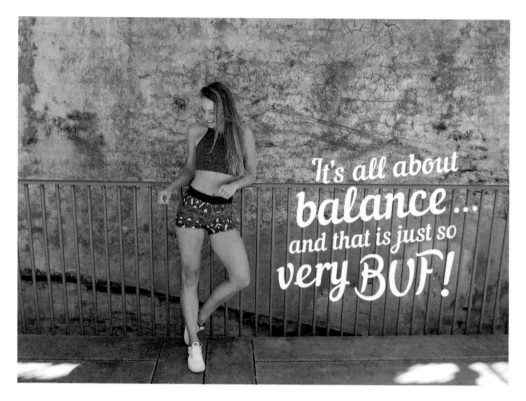

» Choose healthier versions of your favourite grains and snack foods

These days the term 'wholefoods' is used a lot, but what does it really mean?

We at BUF Girls often use the word 'traditional' in place of 'whole' to help our clients understand, because really, all a wholefood is is a food that is as close to its original state as possible. Wholefoods are not treated with preservatives, additives, colours, artificial sweeteners, added sugars, salts, man-made trans fats and extreme heats.

Your metabolism runs more efficiently on food in its natural form, or at least very close to it. Eat a meal of fish, steamed greens and sweet potato with a little organic butter and guess what happens? Your body will use all that protein and quality carbohydrate to fuel your body. It will use the good fats for brain power and to keep your metabolism happy. It will soak up all the vitamins and nutrients in the meal to keep you healthy and energised. It will use the fibre and water from the vegetables to process the meal, while the live enzymes will help your digestion fire up.

But eat a packet of chips and it's just empty calories, without the benefits. Not only that, the unhealthy fats, salts and maybe even sugar can create inflammation, making your body work overtime to get back to a state of good health.

The less processed, packaged food you eat, and the more natural foods, the better will be your health, waistline, happiness and energy. As a bonus, all the fibre, protein and other good stuff will help curb your cravings.

You don't have to avoid everything in a packet. Some tinned foods, frozen veggies, dairy products, breads, low-sugar mueslis and condiments can be great additions to your wholefood diet. But when it comes to junk and convenience foods, make sure you choose wisely. Shop more around the outside of the supermarket, where all the fresh food is displayed, rather than in the middle aisles where the lollies, muesli bars, baked goods, crackers and long-life products hang out.

TO GRAIN OR NOT TO GRAIN, THAT IS THE QUESTION

There are countless experts who will tell you grains are unhealthy. There are many others who will argue the opposite. Our opinion is that whether grains are good for you or not depends on one very important thing: you! Every body is unique and what works for one person doesn't necessarily work for another. If you're curious, we'd suggest trying a low-grain, gluten-free diet for a while (anywhere from 1 to 6 weeks is a good start) and paying close attention to how you feel and the ways your body and mindset change.

Keeping a 'food & mood' diary, in which you record what you eat at each meal and how you felt in the few hours following it, is a great way to keep track. If the outcome is a less bloated, leaner, more energetic you, then you know you're on to a good thing.

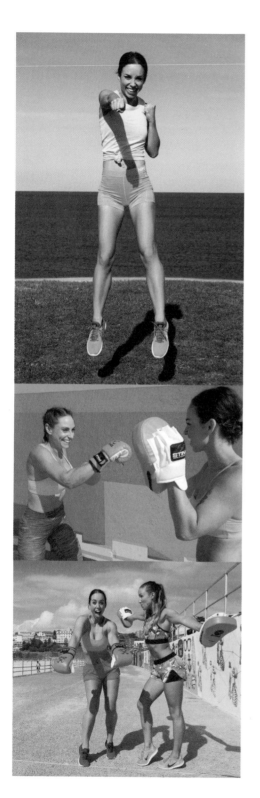

On the flip side, if you find you feel better with a few more carbs on your plate, cool. The important part is listening to what your body is telling you.

Experimentation and staying curious is what this week is all about, and we're here to help you broaden your foodie horizons and get some fresh ideas on your plate.

WHOLEGRAINS AND SLOW-RELEASE CARBOHYDRATES FOR THE WIN

So, we've established that fast-release carbohydrates like sugar, lollies, syrups, honey, fruit juices, white bread, energy bars, crackers, biscuits and baked goods destabilise your blood sugar levels, putting you on the cravings train and leaving you at risk of harming your health.

Slow-release carbohydrates do just the opposite. Wholegrain or vegetable-based foods that are packed with fibre are absorbed slowly and steadily, with the result that your blood sugars don't rise and crash too quickly and your appetite remains steady. As a bonus, they fill you up and keep your appetite hormones happy.

Healthy, fibre-rich wholegrain carbohydrates include foods like dark rye breads and grainy sourdoughs, brown or wild rice, quinoa, oats and steel-cut oats. There are also a lot of vegetable-based slow carbohydrates, like beans and legumes, starchy and non-starchy vegetables and whole fruits, as well as wholegrain and ancient flours.

Here's a handy table that will help you make great choices next time you're craving carbs but want to eat the healthiest version possible:

SWAP THIS GRAIN OR STARCH …	FOR THIS GRAIN OR STARCH …	OR EVEN BETTER …
white bread	grainy or rye bread, traditional chewy sourdough, sprouted breads, wholegrain wraps, grainy gluten-free bread	skip the bread and add more protein, healthy fats or vegetables to your meal
hot chips	roast or baked potatoes	home-baked sweet potato fries, pumpkin chunks or parsnip chips
water crackers, white rice crackers, crisps/chips, corn chips, peanut, soy crackers	plain air-popped popcorn, salted brown rice crackers, sprouted grain crackers, toasted wholegrain flatbread	vegetable sticks (celery, carrot, capsicum, cucumber), sliced fruit
muffin, croissant, biscuit, pastry, banana bread, muesli bar, pre-bought trail mix	a healthy food bar or ball that's low in sugar with minimal ingredients and preservatives. Another option is to reach for a slice of grainy toast topped with nut butter and banana slices.	homemade trail mix with some raw or activated nuts and a few pieces of dried fruit (not much), some apple or banana slices topped with a little nut butter, or make your own BUF treats from this book
refined cereals, high-sugar mueslis, granola, bircher mueslis	low-sugar muesli or high-fibre bran cereals	plain oats, homemade and unsweetened mueslis and granolas, savoury breakfasts
office birthday cake	raw cake made with no refined sugar, or homemade chocolate-dipped strawberries, or a fruit platter with candles on top	give a gift the whole office will remember by starting a tradition of taking the birthday girl or guy out for a half-hour lunchtime walk with the team!
big pasta dishes topped with sauce or meat	lots of vegetables and some quality meat, with half a cup of cooked wholegrain pasta tossed through for texture and some low-sugar sauce or diced tomatoes stirred in	swap the pasta for zoodles and coodles – spiralised zucchini and carrots that look and taste like noodles when cooked!

How to prepare grains healthily

Sprouting, soaking and fermenting your grains are the three healthiest ways to prepare them, allowing your body to more easily digest and absorb the vitamins from them.

Soaking is probably the easiest option for the home cook. All you need to do is rinse your grains, pop them in enough water to cover them, add a squeeze of lemon or a spoonful of vinegar and leave to soak for a minimum of 6–12 hours. Then drain and prepare as you usually would, cooking the grains or putting them in your smoothies or breakfast creations.

How much is too much?

This is individual, depending on your personal energy needs and body goals, but generally half a cup is the right serve of starchy carbohydrates per meal.

WHAT'S THE GO WITH GLUTEN?

Gluten is the name of a protein found naturally in wheat, rye, barley and spelt. Gluten is also added to many processed foods to improve their texture.

There's been a huge trend towards gluten-free eating in recent years, but gluten is not the enemy unless you have Coeliac disease, an auto-immune condition where your immune system reacts abnormally to gluten, causing small bowel damage and inflammation. Other people who may find it beneficial to avoid gluten are those with Irritable Bowel Syndrome. If you suffer from digestive issues, extreme fatigue, gas and bloating, or restlessness or anxiety that seems linked to meal times, your health practitioner can run a few tests to see whether you need to be concerned about Coeliac disease.

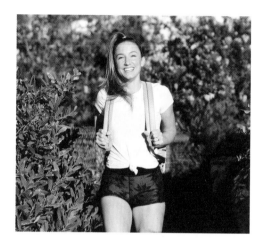

But even if you get the all-clear, you might still be gluten sensitive, so if you're just curious then there's nothing wrong with going G-free for a little while to see how you feel, or at least mixing up your carbohydrate sources to moderate your intake.

Be aware, though, that just because something's gluten free, there's no guarantee it's healthy. In fact, a lot of gluten-free products have added fats, refined starches or sugars to bulk them up and make them taste better.

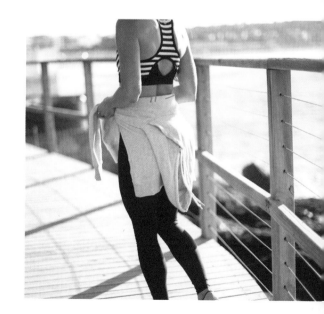

Common foods containing gluten

Wheat, wheat germ, rye, barley, bulgur, couscous, semolina, spelt.

Bread, pasta, baked goods, crackers, pastries, deep-fried foods, sauces, malt-flavoured drinks, mayonnaise, soy and teriyaki sauces, salad dressings, processed meats, egg substitutes, meat substitutes and veggie patties, tabbouleh, sausages, fruit fillings, beer, trail mix, energy bars,

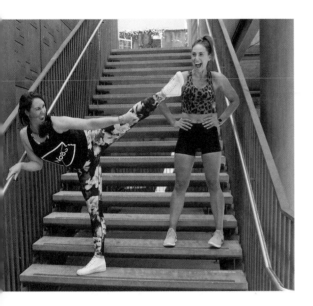

muesli bars, syrups, oats and oat brans that aren't labelled as 'gluten free', vodka, instant hot drinks, some chocolates, some natural colours and flavours, some packaged soups and pre-made meals.

Some gluten-free foods

The obvious ones are vegetables, fruits and animal products like meat, eggs, fish and most dairy foods. But when it comes to gluten-free grains or grain substitutes, as well as condiments, try these on for size: rice, quinoa, buckwheat, millet, amaranth, uncontaminated oats, sorghum, teff, legumes, beans, hummus, coconut flour, chickpea flour, almond flour, mustard,

horseradish, tapenade, salsa, coconut aminos, and apple cider vinegar.

HOW OFTEN SHOULD YOU BE EATING BREAD?

Time for the BIG question, and we know it's one dear to every girl's heart: just how much is too much when it comes to bread?

Bread is one of those basic, satisfying foods that makes for a great base for just about anything, from poached eggs to pizza and everything in between. We would never want to give bread up ourselves, so we won't pretend you need to either, but when it comes to how often you should include bread in your diet, keep in mind that just because you *can* doesn't mean you always *should*. Bread is a very energy-dense product with few nutrients and plenty of gluten, and a lot of brands you'll find at the supermarket are made from refined flour and oils. That's a combination that adds up to one pretty inflammatory and high-calorie food choice, so moderation is key.

Almost every modern disease is arguably caused or affected by inflammation of some sort, and too much can result in an impaired immune system, chronic illness, weight gain (or an inability to shed those final few kilograms) and premature ageing, among other things. With this in mind, it's a good idea to put bread in the 'sometimes food' basket, or rotate your menu and have a break from it when you can by using alternatives.

No one suggested serving size is right for everyone, but 1–2 pieces per day is plenty as a guide, and there's nothing wrong with cutting it out altogether and including more vegetables and other nutrient-packed foods instead if you're keen to lean down a bit.

PACKAGED DOESN'T ALWAYS MEAN PROCESSED

We know the healthiest foods are those that either grew or walked on the earth and are consumed whole, or prepared as simply as possible. Fresh vegetables, fruits, nuts and seeds, beans and legumes, properly prepared wholegrains, wild and sustainably caught seafood, grass-fed meats and pressed plant oils, like olive and coconut oil ... eat a diet full of these foods and it's hard to go wrong. But don't be led into believing that all packaged and processed foods are nasty. Some are downright healthy and fine to include in your healthy BUF life. In fact, a few long-life foods stashed in your fridge, freezer and pantry can be absolute saviours in a tight spot and stop you reaching for takeaway foods when you land home from work late and hungry.

Here's our list of the best 'processed' supermarket buys:

Frozen vegetables More vegetables is a good thing, no matter how you get them in, but the good news is the frozen variety are right up there on the 'angelic foods' scale.

Frozen fruits We love that you can find wild-grown organic fruits in the freezer aisle that would be impossible to get fresh otherwise!

Microwaveable rice Of course, preparing your rice from scratch by soaking, rinsing and cooking it is always best, but we're busy women and often that's just not a practical option! The quick-cook bags of microwaveable rice you find on supermarket shelves aren't too bad, as long as you go for the plain brown, wild or basmati varieties, without added vegetable oils or 'special flavours'. It's always better to remove the rice from the plastic pouch and put it in a bowl before you zap it, to avoid eating plastic toxins with your meal.

Tinned beans and tomatoes Beans are rich in nutrients and fibre, as well as being very filling and pretty low in calories, while tomatoes make a great base for many recipes. Tinned beans and tomatoes are fairly healthy if they haven't had salt added to them and don't come in toxic packaging, so look for those 'no salt added' and 'BPA free' labels, then stock up and use them in soups, salads, stir-fries and Mediterranean-inspired dishes, or take mini bean tins with you for simple snacks at work. All varieties are great for you!

Tinned fish Salmon, mackerel and sardines in particular are incredibly healthy. Look for wild-caught fish, packed in spring water or olive oil.

Dried or dehydrated foods As long as they're free of added oils, sugars and salts, dried fruit and semi-dried vegetable products can make great meal savers.

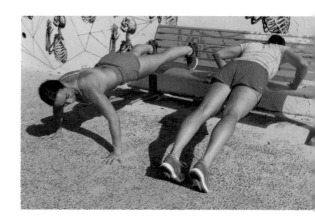

Fermented and pickled foods Sauerkraut, kimchi, pickles and olives all provide digestive and health benefits, so these are definitely worth picking up and including in your salads, on your plate, or as snacks.

Condiments We're not talking tomato sauce, barbecue sauce or sweet chilli sauce here – these are all up to 50 per cent sugar! Instead, reach for mustards,

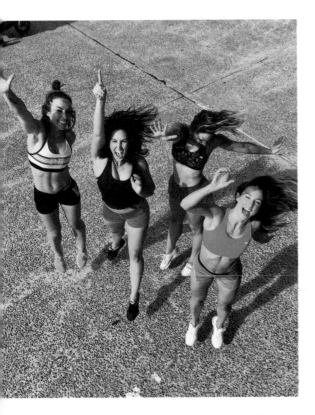

chilli sauce with no sugar added, and pre-mixed blends of salt-free spices. Choose traditional, simple condiments that are low in sugar, salt and oil.

Fresh dips Pre-made hummus, babaganoush and guacamole can be super-healthy so long as they contain good oils like olive oil, or no oil at all. Check the ingredients. There are also some really cool little packs of mushy avocado in supermarkets now, containing no other ingredients at all!

Dark chocolate Train your tastebuds to come over to the dark side! Chocolate is loaded with antioxidants and nutrients that can positively affect your health, but eating brands high in sugar will reduce the benefits, so just check the nutrition panel for brands with 5–10 g of sugar or less per 100 g.

THE BIGGEST SWAP OF ALL: SWAP DIETING FOR A HEALTHY LIFESTYLE

Let's get one thing clear. For most women, permanent weight loss is simply the side effect of a healthy body.

If you have a history of drastic dieting, unhealthy eating habits, a sedentary lifestyle, health issues or medications, it can take a little bit longer for your body to reduce inflammation, find balance and let go of the extra weight. That's totally normal and very much okay. Try to stay patient, stick with the basic principles of eating for optimum health, moving more, using stress-reduction techniques, learning to cook healthy food and continuing to educate yourself on health and nutrition. Even better, find a fun, healthy, supportive community to be part of that inspires you and lifts you up every day.

It can be hard to be patient and not fall for the quick fixes, but instead of focusing on all the things you don't like about your body, try acknowledging all the really positive actions you're taking every single day, each one making you just that little bit healthier. If you wake up with more energy, celebrate it. Feeling less fatigued after a full day of work? Chalk that up as a win. Went for a walk every day this week after lunch and avoided afternoon burnout? Get excited about that new habit! Sleeping better? That's a sign you're on the right path!

Take a moment to celebrate those little wins and know they're steps on the path to finally feeling (b)eautiful in your body, (u)nstoppable on your path to great health, and creating a (f)earless mindset that will set you up for life.

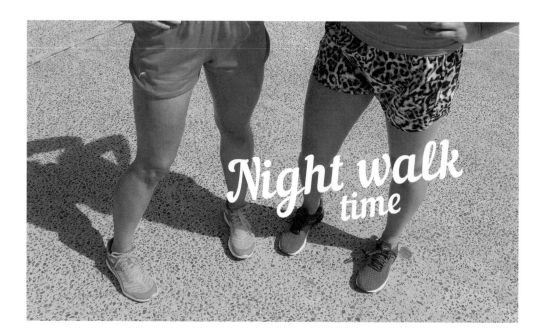

Night walk time

» Add 'night walks' to your schedule

If you do nothing else, this one simple movement habit can totally change your health, fitness and body shape. Even better, it can add spark to your closest relationships.

All you have to do is gather your partner, dog, sister or housemate, or just load up a good playlist, and take off for a walk right after dinner's finished. Kids in particular LOVE these, and after a few evenings of strolling the streets with you, they will be chanting, 'Night walk time!' before you've even put the plates away.

The walk itself can be anything from a 5-minute stroll around the block to a 15-minute power walk, or a longer 30–60 minute waltz under the stars on a summer's night.

The benefits of taking a night walk are many, but here are our favourites ...

- Your meal digests better and you'll experience less bloating.
- You avoid going straight from dinner table to screen, whether that's a TV, computer or phone.
- It's a great way to wind down for sleep.
- More time moving means less time mindlessly snacking on the couch.
- A brisk walk after meals helps shed belly fat and improves nutrient absorption.
- It stimulates your metabolism and lowers your blood sugar levels.
- A night walk is an incredible ritual to help you connect with the ones you love, minus technology and plus a whole lot of creative conversation.

» Harness the powerful connection between food and mood

There's a super-powerful connection between food and mood. Learning to harness those powers for good can change the entire way you approach your day, so read up, eat up and feel UP!

For ongoing happiness and motivation ... eat 'smart' carbs Carbs contain tryptophan, a non-essential amino acid that helps serotonin (the happy hormone) synthesise in the brain, improving your mood. Reach for fruits, vegetables, beans and legumes, and wholegrains.

To calm anxiety and boost focus ... eat oily fish and walnuts Omega 3s may help protect against depression and anxiety. They also help kick your brain into gear, so eat up on busy work days. Vegetarian? Avocado, flaxseeds and coconut or olive oils should do the trick.

To kick anger ... sip green tea Green tea contains theanine, which calms you and helps you maintain clear concentration.

Cranky and hungry ... eat sliced apple or pear, plus nut butter Quick energy from the apple and sustained energy from the nut butter makes this the perfect hunger-busting afternoon snack if you've accidentally slipped into your fave pair of cranky-pants.

Sluggish ... eat spinach salad, or steamed leafy greens Foods packed with folic acid help your body improve blood flow to the brain, which sharpens concentration.

Need to fire up for a big day ... eat meat or fish, plus nuts for breakfast Small portions of these two foods will stimulate the production of neurotransmitters responsible for waking you up, sharpening your focus and putting you in a 'can do' mood.

Stressed ... eat dark chocolate, almonds, artichoke or kidney beans Packed with magnesium, which has mild muscle-relaxing qualities, these foods can help reduce stress and improve mood.

Exhausted ... eat pumpkin seeds, bok choy, legumes, sea vegetables or red meat If you don't have enough iron in your blood, exhaustion can set in pretty quickly. Stock up on iron-rich foods to avoid plummeting energy levels.

Lethargic ... drink a green smoothie A heavy meal can often make you feel sluggish, so if you're looking for an energy hit without the drag, load your blender up with greens, blend and go!

A quick list of mood-draining foods

- **Processed soy foods** – tofu, soy milk.
- **Diet soft drink** – it may have no sugar, but it's full to the brim with mood-altering chemicals.
- **Refined sugar** – gives you an instant energy boost, but the crash that follows can bring a blue mood with it.
- **Coffee overload** – stop at 1 for max energy.
- **Trans fats** – recent studies show that these unhealthy fats (found in most processed and deep-fried foods and a lot of commercially baked goods) are strongly linked to depression.

TOP TIPS 'n' TAKEAWAYS

» Choose the healthiest version of the food you're craving.

» Grains can be a nourishing, filling food if you understand how to make the right choices.

» Slow-release carbohydrates will give you lasting energy, without the crash.

» Vegetables, fruits, nuts, seeds and dairy products are all grain-free sources of carbohydrates.

» You don't have to stop eating your favourite snacks, just swap them for a slightly healthier version. Get creative and stay curious!

» Gluten is a protein found in wheat, rye, barley and oats. For some people, gluten is easily digestible and doesn't affect their overall health. However, for a growing number of people, gluten can lead to niggling health issues they'd rather live without. It's worth cutting down, or removing gluten from your diet every now and then, to give your body a break.

» Properly prepare your wholegrains by rinsing and soaking them.

» Take a walk after dinner – it's a powerful weight-loss and health-boosting tool.

» Women need carbohydrates to keep hormones balanced and fertility optimal, so don't go without, just swap the refined carbs for unrefined ones.

WEEK THREE
MEAL PLAN

	Breakfast	*Lunch*	*Dinner*
MONDAY	Coconut Porridge PAGE 108	Pearl Barley and Bean Salad PAGE 160	Mushroom and Cauliflower Pizza PAGE 202
TUESDAY	Fried Eggs with Almond Butter Greens PAGE 110	Kale, Fennel and Apple Salad PAGE 152	Baked Eggplant and Lentils PAGE 178
WEDNESDAY	Green Smoothie Bowl PAGE 113	Roast Veggie Patties PAGE 170	Mushroom and Chicken Pesto Stacks PAGE 204
THURSDAY	Quinoa Cacao Muesli PAGE 126	Open Chicken Sanga PAGE 158	Cumin-spiced Meatballs with Carrot 'Pasta' PAGE 192
FRIDAY	Toast Toppers PAGE 124	Rainbow Abundance Bowl PAGE 166	Kale and Mushroom Rice with Chicken PAGE 196

Snack options
» PARSNIP CHIPS (PAGE 243)
» SUPERFOOD TRAIL MIX (PAGE 246)
» BLISS BALLS (PAGE 233)

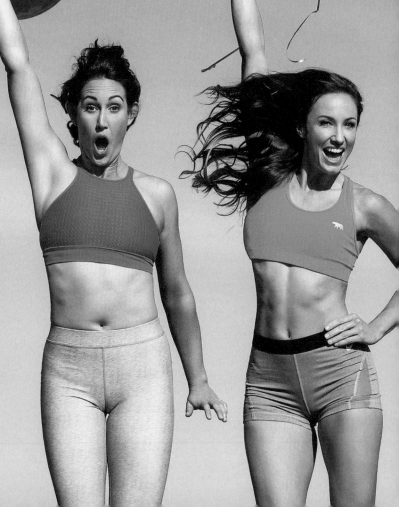

Banish the Bloat

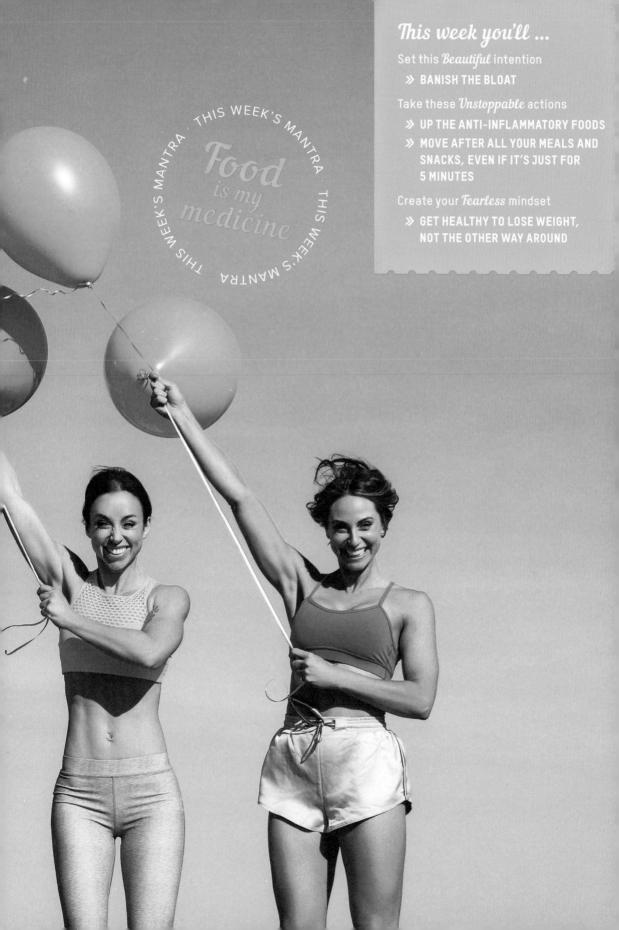

This week you'll ...

Set this *Beautiful* intention

» **BANISH THE BLOAT**

Take these *Unstoppable* actions

» **UP THE ANTI-INFLAMMATORY FOODS**
» **MOVE AFTER ALL YOUR MEALS AND SNACKS, EVEN IF IT'S JUST FOR 5 MINUTES**

Create your *Fearless* mindset

» **GET HEALTHY TO LOSE WEIGHT, NOT THE OTHER WAY AROUND**

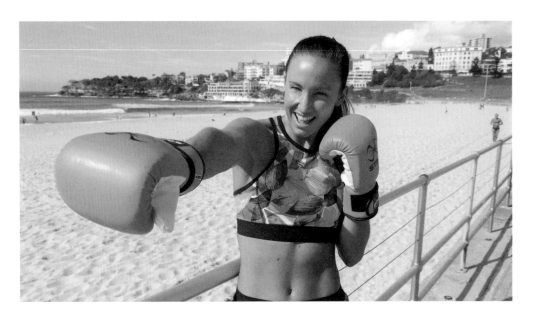

» *Banish the bloat*

Most women experience bloating from time to time. It's pretty normal for it to happen occasionally, and kind of unavoidable at certain times of the month. Even if you're one of the lucky ones who never suffers from a bloated belly after meals, this week's anti-inflammatory food plan can still help calm your nerves, reduce stress, relieve depression, make your skin glow, reduce pain in your joints, help you recover better after tough workouts, and lighten the load on your liver to make getting lean simpler.

Embracing anti-inflammatory eating may also help prevent diseases such as diabetes and cardiovascular disease, help to improve existing inflammatory conditions (like auto-immune diseases, polycystic ovary syndrome, arthritis, asthma, endometriosis, acne and eczema) and balance your hormones to support healthy ovulation and fertility.

This is the week of your program we lovingly refer to as 'happy body week', although some of the girls who've gone through it have jokingly renamed it 'flat tummy week' because it made them feel so much more comfortable. It's all about feeding your body the kind of foods that help it to heal, balance and detoxify naturally, and of course to banish bloating as much as possible.

We'll also take a look at how stress and lack of sleep affect digestion, mindset and body shape, and what you can do to flip the switch.

Sounds like something worth doing, right?

» *Up the anti-inflammatory foods*

Inflammation is believed to be one of the root causes of many imbalances and stress responses in the body, so it makes good sense that shifting to foods that reduce inflammation responses can help to prevent or improve certain conditions, and at the very least help to calm your nerves and ease stress.

WHAT IS INFLAMMATION ANYWAY?

There are two kinds of inflammation in your body, and, a bit like cholesterol, one's the good guy and one's the bad guy.

Acute inflammation: 'the good guy'

This is the kind of inflammation that happens after an injury like a sprained ankle, burn or cut. It's local, temporary, and without it your wounds wouldn't heal. Your body uses swelling to drive proteins, white blood cells and antibodies into the injured area and start reconstructing tissue and blood vessels.

Acute inflammation is also what allows your muscles to grow and change when you start an exercise program. This is why you don't want to take anti-inflammatory pills to deal with muscle pain after a workout (at least, not unless you're really desperate!) – it might just reverse the effects of all your hard work. You're better off going for a long, slow walk and getting fresh blood pumping through your body to help things return to normal quickly.

Chronic inflammation: 'the bad guy'

This is sometimes called persistent, low-grade inflammation and usually creeps into your life slowly, so you may not notice anything amiss at first.

Chronic inflammation usually begins when your body reacts to a particular food or other unhealthy lifestyle choice, or to emotional stress, or to a bacteria or virus. The result is a bit like a whole army showing up to go to war against just one person. Basically, your body overreacts to a threat it thinks is bigger than it is, and if you keep doing/eating the things triggering this response, the swelling and biochemical onslaught can just go on and on, creating constant inflammation inside your body. Not only does this cause suffering but other goals are also put on hold. **Muscle growth and fat loss can be stopped in their tracks when chronic inflammation is present in the body.**

FIRING UP YOUR BODY'S FAT-BURNING FURNACE

Did you know your liver is the major fat-burning organ in your body? Yep, your hardworking liver not only regulates fat metabolism and converts excess carbohydrates and proteins into fatty acids and triglyceride, which are then stored as adipose (fat) tissue, it can also pump excessive fat out of the body through your bile into the small intestine, where it is excreted as waste.

This means a healthy liver is critical for weight management because, if your liver isn't regulating fat metabolism efficiently, weight gain quickly occurs around your tummy area and becomes tough to shift. A healthy liver also plays a key role in

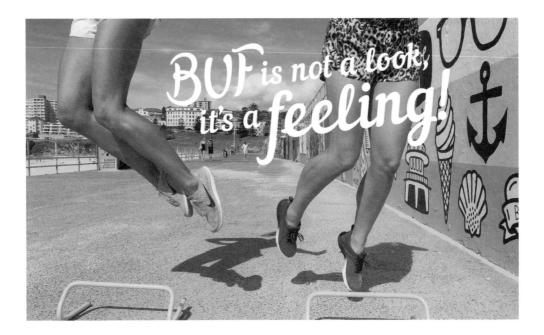

relieving digestive issues like gas, bloating and constipation, while regulating blood sugar levels to reduce sugar cravings, fatigue and fuzzy thinking.

If you don't consistently choose healthy foods that support liver health, you not only end up feeling sluggish, you can also develop a 'fatty liver', which is a condition where your liver stops burning fat and starts storing it rapidly, becoming enlarged with deposits of fatty tissue. When this happens, you can't lose weight at all until you have addressed the accumulated liver fat. Then weight loss will become easier again.

The scary thing is, the first signs that your liver is starting to struggle are raised liver enzymes and inflammation in the body, which are only things you can find out by getting a blood test, so it's often something that goes unnoticed for a long time.

This is one situation where prevention is definitely a better option than trying to reverse the effects of high inflammation in your body, or worse, fatty liver

disease. That's why this week is all about understanding how to reduce inflammation and keep your fat-burning furnace firing strongly!

RECOGNISE THESE EATING PATTERNS?

We've all done it – wake up to cereal with a liberal dose of honey and a slice of toast, revel in a warm and comforting mid-morning latte, grab a sandwich in our lunch break, pick up something sweet (and maybe another cup of coffee!) after lunch, hit the office lolly jar to make it through the last few hours of the day, then finish off with a nice glass of vino (or two) and some takeaway or an easy-to-make dish of pasta and sauce when you get home. Oh, and ice-cream or chocolate before bed, of course.

If you're eating and drinking this way consistently, chances are you're already stressing your liver and creating unwanted inflammation in your body. As your major detoxification and fat-burning hub, you need your liver to be in top working order.

So what's on and off the menu this week?

EAT THIS	REDUCE THAT	WHY?
Dark, leafy greens like spinach, kale, cabbage and collard greens, plus cruciferous vegetables like broccoli, asparagus, cauliflower, bok choy and Brussels sprouts	If you get bloated easily, avoid eating your veggies raw. Instead, gently steam, sauté or bake them to help your body digest them without extra gas	The veggies pack a nutrient punch, reduce inflammation and support healthy digestion, while cooking them a little minimises gas and bloating
Dark-skinned fruits like berries and red grapes, cherries, pomegranate, tomatoes and oranges	Limit higher-sugar fruits like banana, mango, melon and dried varieties to one serve per day	Dark fruits are anti-inflammatory and packed with antioxidants that help prevent cell damage
Oily fish like salmon, sardines, mackerel, herring, trout, anchovies, or a good-quality fish oil supplement	Industrial-made trans fats found in packaged and deep-fried foods, as well as fried baked goods like doughnuts	Good fats are incredibly powerful for your health, while man-altered trans fats will destroy it quicker than you can say 'death by doughnut'
Plant-based fats and oils like avocado and avocado oil, olives and olive oil, coconut flesh and coconut oil, tree nuts and tree nut oils (almonds, cashews, brazils, macadamias, etc.), whole seeds and chia seeds	Processed vegetable oils like sunflower, soy, safflower and blended vegetable oils	Natural, cold-pressed oils are the product of minimal processing, while vegetable oils are generally extracted under high heat and using chemicals, making them much less health-friendly
A little real, organic butter	Margarine or spreads with partially-hydrogenated oils	A little organic butter is good for the soul and your waistline, but the oils in other spreads fall into the 'nasty fats' category
Small serves (100 g max per serve) of good-quality, ideally organic or grass-fed/free-range meats like beef, lamb, chicken and turkey	Processed meats like sausages, bacon, deli meats and packaged/long-life meats	Processed meats with lots of fat and additives, which means they last for months without going off? Erm, no thanks.

EAT THIS	REDUCE THAT	WHY?
Small amounts of hard cheeses or soft cheeses like goat cheese or ricotta	Processed cheeses and cheese spreads	When it comes to dairy, the less meddled with, the better!
Small serves of full-fat dairy, like plain Greek yoghurt and organic whole milk, or dairy alternatives like coconut milk/yoghurt and nut milks (choose ones with less than 5 g sugar per 100 g)	Sugary fruit yoghurts and skim dairy products	Fruit yoghurts often contain up to 7 teaspoons of sugar in one small tub – eek! And skim products don't have the health benefits and satiate your hunger like full-fat ones do.
High-fibre, slow-release carbohydrates like beans and legumes, oats, quinoa, brown or wild rice, sweet potatoes and pumpkin, beetroot and corn	Refined carbohydrates like white bread, pasta, baked goods, cereal, sugar, syrups, sweets and sugary chocolate	So many reasons ... let's just say this is one of the most important things to take away from this entire book!
Herbs and spices like chilli, basil, thyme, turmeric, ginger, oregano and garlic	Pre-seasoned food and seasoning mixes	It's crazy how much salt pre-seasoned food and mixes can contain – and that means bloating is almost inevitable! Spices speed up your metabolism and nourish your body, so they're a much better choice.
Olive oil, fresh squeezes of citrus and vinegars	Bottled sauces and salad dressings	Pre-made sauces and dressings are loaded with sugar, salts and preservatives. Go for the good stuff instead.
Water, herbal teas, sparkling water, chai and turmeric chai, dandelion root tea	Alcohol and caffeine (yowch, but it's important to reduce these this week!)	Dehydration is a major cause of bloating and a potent energy zapper. Alcohol and caffeine are major contributors to dehydration.
Digestion saviours like natural yoghurt, kefir, sauerkraut, kimchi and bone broth	Unfermented dairy and soy products	Fermented foods come loaded with enzymes that fuel digestion and gut health, whereas too much unfermented dairy and soy products can cause bloating for some people, and sluggish digestion in others

EMBRACING HEALTHY FATS

Here's how to get this right:

EMBRACE olive oil, avocado and avocado oil, nuts and seeds, oily fish, coconut oil, bone broth, chia seeds

ENJOY IN MODERATION meat and dairy products

AVOID all deep-fried foods, crisps, packaged biscuits, fried crackers

We've often thought about how great it would be if dietary fats weren't actually called 'fats', because the name tends to scare women away from eating this incredibly important macronutrient.

So many people still worry that eating fat will make them fat; it's an assumption that seems hard to change. Fat actually plays an important role in regulating appetite, hormones, energy production and metabolism, and it ticks all the anti-inflammatory boxes too.

We'd go so far as to say that eating the right kind of fat is one of the best ways ever to signal your body to release and burn stored fat. This is because dietary fat activates the fat-burning pathways through the liver, which encourage your body to release the stored fat around your belly, thighs, butt and arms (this is called subcutaneous fat, or the fat that sits just under your skin), and also because dietary fat helps keep insulin levels low.

Insulin is the hormone responsible for shuttling the sugar from carbohydrates and, to some extent, from proteins, out of your bloodstream to where it's needed – usually to your muscles and organs for use as energy. But insulin also *triggers* the storage of fat in adipose tissue, so while insulin is in your blood, you literally can't burn stored fat. So, eating more carbohydrates, particularly the refined and sugary kind, means less time in fat-burning mode and more fat accumulation in your body.

Eating fat also triggers the release of another important hormone, called leptin, which triggers feelings of fullness and stops you from wanting to snack all the time. As a bonus, fat allows you to better absorb fat-soluble vitamins such as A, D, E and K. Consequently, you get more benefit from the ingredients in a salad if you add some olive oil or avocado, or sprinkle on a few seeds.

But here comes the catch ... to get all the benefits, you've got to eat the right kind of fats. Bye bye deep-fried chips!

While healthy fats will help you get lean, boost energy, drive hormone production and keep your brain all fired up, others are best consumed in moderation, and the industrial-made kind will wreak absolute havoc on your body.

Fibre is important

Next we need to discuss the importance of fibre. It can help regulate digestion and reduce inflammation – both outcomes that get a big tick during banish bloating week.

Your body needs two types of fibre: soluble and insoluble.

Soluble fibre mixes with water to form a gel, which slows digestion. It helps the body better absorb nutrients, and may also lower total cholesterol and LDL, or 'bad' cholesterol. This kind of fibre can be found in foods like nuts, seeds, beans, lentils, oat bran and barley.

Insoluble fibre helps your digestive system run more efficiently. It adds bulk to your poop, which helps prevent constipation. The best sources of insoluble fibre are vegetables, fruits, wholegrains, beans and legumes.

What causes bloating?

Any of these things may be happening when you experience bloating:

- hormonal fluctuation
- the pooling of liquid, gas or solid contents in parts of the gut
- constipation or the slow movement of contents through the intestine
- weak muscles in the abdominal wall
- a diaphragm muscle that contracts when it should relax

There are definitely a few dietary factors that can make bloating worse, or more common than it needs to be, including:

- eating in a stressed or rushed state
- eating too much in one sitting
- food intolerances
- poorly digested sugars, usually from lactose or fructose intolerance
- artificial sugar intake
- changes in gut bacteria, perhaps after a course of medication or antibiotics following a bacterial or viral infection, or after a period of high stress or travel
- a medical condition, such as Irritable Bowel Syndrome or a gluten allergy
- eating too many raw foods
- eating too many raw nuts
- eating fruit, chocolate or other sugars directly after a meal

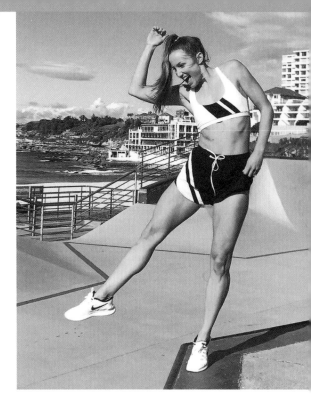

HOW TO REDUCE BLOATING INCIDENCES

Meal-time bloating

- Reduce portion sizes
- Start your meal with foods alive with enzymes – salad, bone broth, fermented foods
- Don't eat sweets or fruit directly after your main meals
- Go for a gentle 15-minute walk after meals
- Choose to eat anti-inflammatory foods
- Don't overdo the raw veggies and nuts
- Avoid heavy saturated and trans fats, but add some healthy fats
- Don't overdo the grains
- Avoid drinking water within 15 minutes of meal times – it can dilute digestive enzymes
- Consider eliminating dairy products and gluten for a few weeks to see if that helps at all
- Talk to your health professional if symptoms persist or worsen. He/she may suggest digestive enzymes, probiotics or further tests.

Random bloating

- Try peppermint oil capsules – they're pretty amazing!
- Consider breathing techniques or meditation to reduce stress
- Exercise regularly to improve abdominal wall muscle tone and help clear gas
- Stay hydrated with 8–10 glasses of water or herbal teas each day
- Avoid carbonated drinks and chewing gum
- Take a good-quality magnesium supplement

GOOD GUT HEALTH

Prebiotics, probiotics and a healthy gut

Prebiotics and probiotics are both really important for your gut health. Here's what they do:

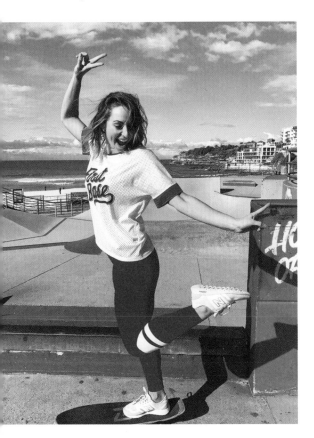

Prebiotics are a special form of starchy dietary fibre that resist digestion in the gastrointestinal tract and are instead metabolised by your gut bacteria, effectively acting as a fertiliser for all the good bacteria in your gut, feeding it and nourishing it. Prebiotics are incredibly helpful for several chronic disorders of the gut and can help calm inflammation, but are also a really important part of everyday gut health. Prebiotics are found in a lot of high fibre vegetables and some grains, like under-ripe bananas, cold potato, rolled oats, berries, onions and garlic, artichokes, beans and lentils.

Probiotics are live bacteria created from lactic acid fermentation of foods. Probiotics can help to replenish your healthy gut bacteria, and it's a good idea to have at least one serve of them per day. Find them in natural foods like plain yoghurt and kefir, sauerkraut, kimchi, cultured butter, naturally preserved olives and pickles, as well as kombucha (check to make sure you're choosing a low-sugar brand). Of course, you can also get probiotics in the form of pills. Ingesting live bacteria in any of these forms can be helpful for maintaining a healthy gut, or replacing bacteria destroyed by a course of antibiotics or a stomach bug. There are hundreds of different species available and unless you have an in-depth gut screen, it can be hard to know exactly what you need, so mix up your sources as often as you can.

What is bone broth and can it improve gut health?

We're not nutritionists or scientists, so we really can't give you a solid thumbs up on this, but we can tell you that bone broth, which is a stock made from boiling animal bones and cartilage, contains an incredible number of amino acids and minerals, as well as collagen, gelatin, glucosamine and a few other things that have been proven to be very anti-inflammatory and healing to the gut.

There seems to be a lot of evidence supporting bone broth as a healing food, particularly for conditions like leaky gut or auto-immune disease, and on a personal level we've found it great for decreasing both bloating *and* cravings. In fact, we challenge you to reach for a warm mug of bone broth next time you have a 3 pm choccy craving and see how much better you feel!

Bone broth is easy enough to make if you have the time, but if you prefer the easy option (erm, *we* do!) there are ready-made, take-anywhere concentrates available online.

Will reducing alcohol help?

As we discussed in Week Two, drinking less alcohol is a really great habit to get into. A huge percentage of alcohol metabolism happens in the liver, putting pressure on your best fat-burning, sugar-regulating organ. This is why a lot of heavy drinkers end up with liver issues.

Alcohol also increases inflammation in your body, while simultaneously increasing your appetite and decreasing your willpower for abstaining from other pro-inflammatory foods. Before you know it, you've had the wine *and* the crisps *and* the biscuits.

Give your gut a break

One of the simplest things you can do to give your digestive system a break and reduce bloating is to provide a decent amount of rest time for your gut on a regular basis.

Try leaving roughly 12 hours between dinner and breakfast – we've found this is a really simple and achievable path to feeling lighter and less bloated for most people.

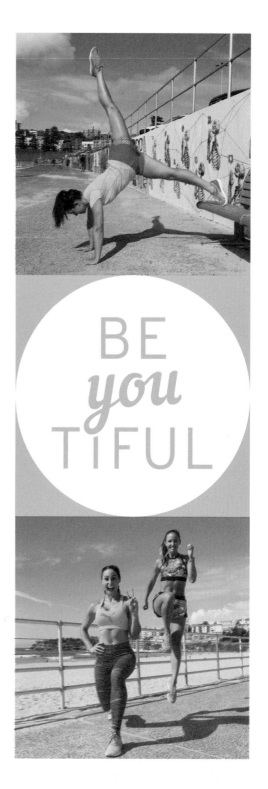

» *Move after your meals*

Taking a walk after your meals could just be one of the best tricks ever in the fat-loss and feel-better books. This one simple action lowers blood sugar levels, encourages your muscles to use up the energy from the food you've just eaten and helps your body to restore balance. Physical activity also aids digestion by giving your insides a gentle massage, activating digestive enzymes and stimulating the nervous, hormone and muscular systems.

Don't do anything too rigorous – you don't want your body to slip out of that sweet 'rest and digest' zone and into 'fight or flight' mode. The best options are mild forms of exercise, like taking a walk or a bike ride, or standing up and down from the couch 10 times during every ad break of your favourite TV show.

Gentle stretching or yoga poses that stimulate digestion (Google this topic for some winners) are a good idea, too, or if you really can't afford the time then even doing a little deep breathing can be a help, as lots of muscles are used when you practise conscious breath work.

This week, be disciplined in doing a minimum of 5 minutes of movement after every meal or snack and see how you feel. Here are some easy bloat-banishing exercises:

1   Take a 5-minute walk in the fresh air.

2   Do a 5-minute 'mini intervals' set on a stationary bike: pedal for 8 seconds fast, then 12 seconds slow, a total of 15 times.

3   Google these digestion-aiding yoga poses and do each of them for one minute: Cat-Cow, Garland Pose, Leg-Binding Pose, Wind-Relieving Pose, Reclined Cobbler's Pose.

4   Breathe the bloat away by finding a quiet spot to sit cross-legged, or on a chair, keeping a tall spine. Hold your hands at the level of your throat, with your palms facing each other and your fingers clasped together, creating a tension as if you were pulling your palms apart. Next, inhale as you twist your torso to the left, then exhale as you twist to the right. Continue this action slowly and gently for 3–4 minutes, then sit quietly with your hands in your lap for 1–2 minutes.

5   Grab a skipping rope and turn it over for 5 minutes, or if you don't have a rope, just bounce gently on the spot.

Banish the bloat

» Get healthy to lose weight – not the other way around!

Let's get one thing straight: a healthy body is absolutely crucial for weight loss to occur, particularly weight loss of the long-term, sustainable kind. Where the 'diet industry' fails women is by suggesting weight loss is the path to health, not the other way around.

Let's look at the facts:

- Eating a very low calorie diet can work short-term, but if you've made the change too quickly, it signals your body to go into 'store everything' mode, slowing your metabolism significantly. This means that when you do start eating normally again, the weight often piles back on.

- If you are protein or nutrient deficient, either from undereating in general, or from overeating foods that are not nourishing, that creates stress for your body and eventually leads to weight gain, disease and exhaustion.

- Weight loss that's too speedy can mess with appetite hormones and make you feel really emotional, a combination that eventually leads to bingeing and anxiety.

- Focusing on 'losing weight' is just NOT FUN and feels like punishment.

HOW TO TELL IF YOU'RE TAKING THE RIGHT APPROACH

A really easy way to check in with whether an eating plan is right for you is to ask, 'Could I eat this way every day, for the rest of my life?' Healthy eating and healthy movement should feel sustainable – something you can keep up indefinitely.

That's not to say you shouldn't stay curious and experiment with new ways to eat and move, but before you dive in, consider whether you're doing it because you want to get healthier, or just because you want a quick fix. **Just like fixing your leaky sink with some sticky tape to save the hassle of getting a plumber in, fad diets don't set your body up for long-term success.**

DITCH THE RULES AND SET SOME PRINCIPLES

Rules aren't much fun to follow, and the stricter they are, the more likely you are to rebel or go off the rails. However, set some principles for yourself that you can really own and the natural desire you have is to want to uphold them.

Examples of rules:

- 'I only eat 1200 calories a day max' (don't get us started ...)

- 'I'm paleo and never ever eat any kind of grain' (but they're so yummy!)

- 'I follow the exact same food plan every day' (boring, right?)

- 'I never eat out as I don't know what's in the food' (never?!)

Examples of principles:

- 'I choose to eat the best-quality version of the food I'm craving' (you can still have the choccy, but you'll grab the lower-sugar, antioxidant-packed darker variety)

- 'Eating food in as close to its natural state as possible is important to me because I want to know what I'm putting in my body' (so naturally the rolled oats are more appealing than the chocolate wheat pop thingos)

- 'Fuelling up with nutrient-packed wholefoods helps me perform at my best at work, and leaves me with more energy for my partner/family at the end of the day' (suddenly that apple and handful of nuts is more appealing than the nutritionally empty biscuit, right?)

- 'I'm grateful for the wonderful life I have and want to wake up fresh and focused, so alcohol is an occasional treat rather than something I rely on to get me through the week' (yes, this is all about leaning into your life, rather than checking out!)

- 'I see movement as a gift and an opportunity to connect with myself and/ or others' (and so it is!)

BE FLEXIBLE WITH MEAL PLANS

In this book we've outlined a few different ways you *can* put the recipes we've created for you together in a weekly meal structure, but just because you can doesn't mean you *should*, and it certainly doesn't mean you *must*.

The problem with a meal plan is that no matter how much you want to stick to it, life gets in the way. You get busy, you get social, you get sick, you work late, you go travelling, you get bored, you feel hungry (or you're not hungry when it's time for that scheduled 10 am protein shake), or you just plain don't feel like eating what's on the plan.

Eventually you give up, and then you feel like a failure. But guess what? All those things that 'got in the way of your plan' are actually really normal things – life events that will *keep on* happening no matter how much you wish they wouldn't disrupt your diet schedule.

On the other hand, you might be the kind of person who sticks to the plan *perfectly*. But what happens when your plan comes to an end? Do you just keep repeating it? Or do you look for the next earth-shattering diet trick?

Unless you're an athlete with a specific goal, meal plans are often just not sustainable. You don't have to eat a specific number of grams of meat, nail your macronutrient ratios exactly, count your walnuts or measure out every grain of rice in order to eat better, create a healthy, lean body and feel like the best version of yourself. You just need to keep making small changes that have big impact.

For example:

- If you love cereal and usually eat a packaged muesli with fruit yoghurt for breakfast, improve the health of your meal by making your own muesli and serving it with plain yoghurt and berries.

- If you usually have a large latte when you get to the office, you could lighten the load by ordering a black coffee with a dash of whole milk instead.

- If you usually grab a cheese and salad sandwich from your office café at lunch time, ask them to hold the bread and put all the ingredients into a bowl with a little chicken or salmon instead; in that way you've just replaced one serve of starchy carbs for one serve of metabolism-loving protein.

It's the little, sustainable actions that stick and eventually build into big, healthy habits, which become the building blocks for the important lifestyle principles you love to live by.

So if you do choose to use a meal plan, remember that the goal is always to stop using the meal plan but keep making healthy choices. **Long-term consistency beats short-term perfection every time.**

TOP TIPS 'n' TAKEAWAYS

» Get healthy to lose weight, not the other way around.

» Two in three women experience periodic bloating, so you're not alone.

» An anti-inflammatory diet can help banish the bloat and supercharge your health.

» Learn to listen to your body and choose to eat more of the foods that agree with you and less of those that cause flare-ups.

» A small amount of movement right after your meals, or when you feel the bloating begin, can really help – use our 5-minute bloat banishers.

» Fibre and water are your friends; make sure you invite them to the party.

» Keep your stress levels in check. Modern-day life can have a negative impact on your digestion. Stress comes in many forms – from eating processed foods, from lack of sleep, from too many stimulants or simply from not giving yourself enough time to recover from intense exercise.

» Caffeine and alcohol should be used mindfully and in moderation.

» Healthy fats can help soothe your tummy in the short term and flatten it in the long term.

» Try fermented foods in a tummy crisis and consider whether you're getting enough prebiotic foods every day.

» Seek professional help if you're really struggling with getting your digestion in check.

MEAL PLAN

	Breakfast	*Lunch*	*Dinner*
MONDAY	Failsafe Breakfast Salad PAGE 109	Cucumber 'Fresh As' Salad PAGE 133	Vegetable Tahini Dream PAGE 230
TUESDAY	Pumpkin, Spinach and Feta Breakfast Muffins PAGE 118	Zucchini and Turmeric Soup PAGE 176	Mexican Stuffed Capsicums PAGE 200
WEDNESDAY	Veggie Quinoa Bowl PAGE 120	Avocado and Strawberry Salad PAGE 132	Pan-fried Salmon with Sautéed Greens PAGE 208
THURSDAY	Asparagus Egg Scramble PAGE 101	Pesto Roast Vegetables PAGE 153	Mediterranean Salad PAGE 181
FRIDAY	Glow Juice PAGE 112	Coconut Poached Chicken with Leafy Greens PAGE 148	Turmeric, Cauliflower and Egg Salad PAGE 226

Snack options

» PERFECT 3 PM FIXES (PAGE 246)

» KALE CHIPS (PAGE 242)

» TURMERIC CHAI (PAGE 245)

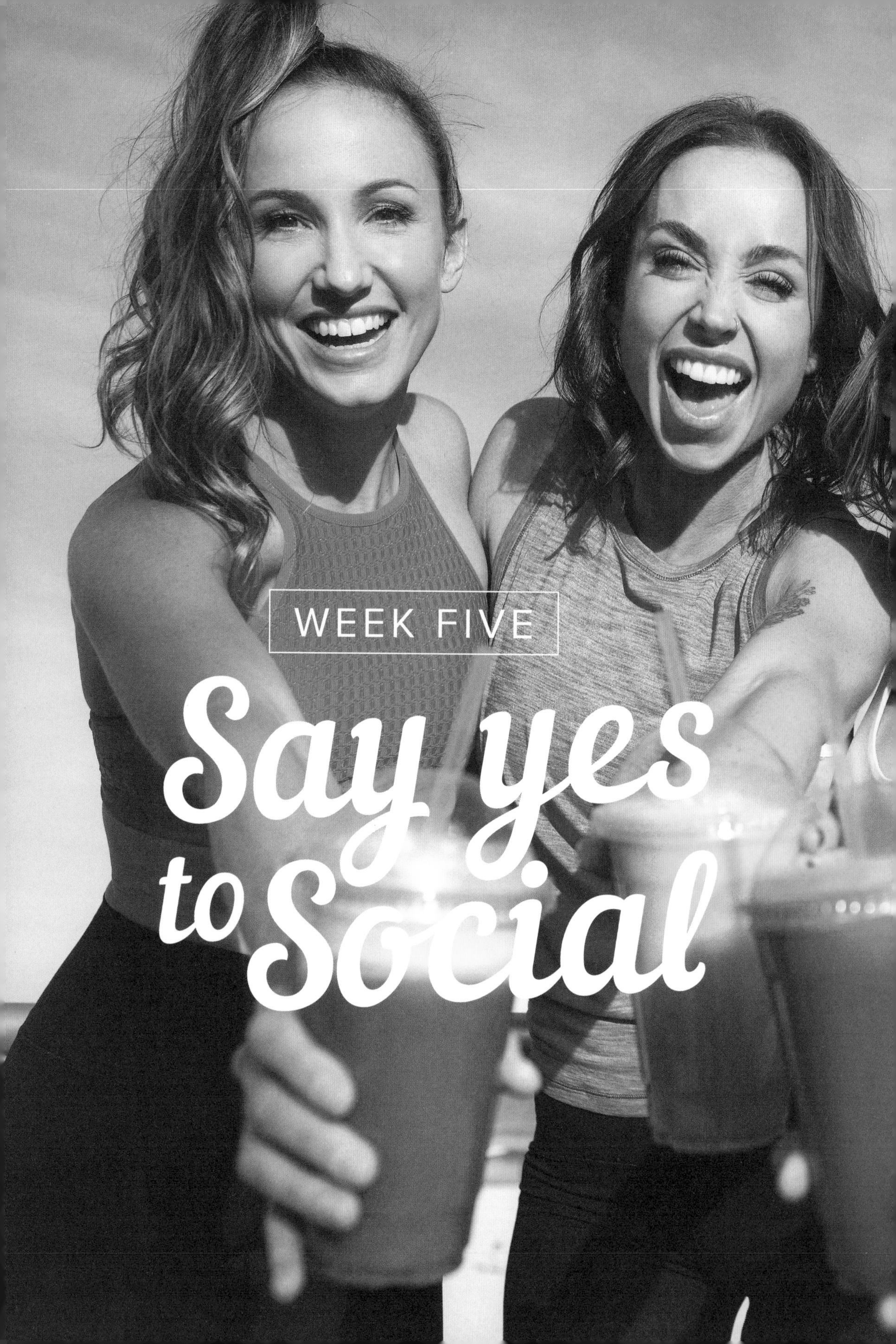

WEEK FIVE

Say yes to Social

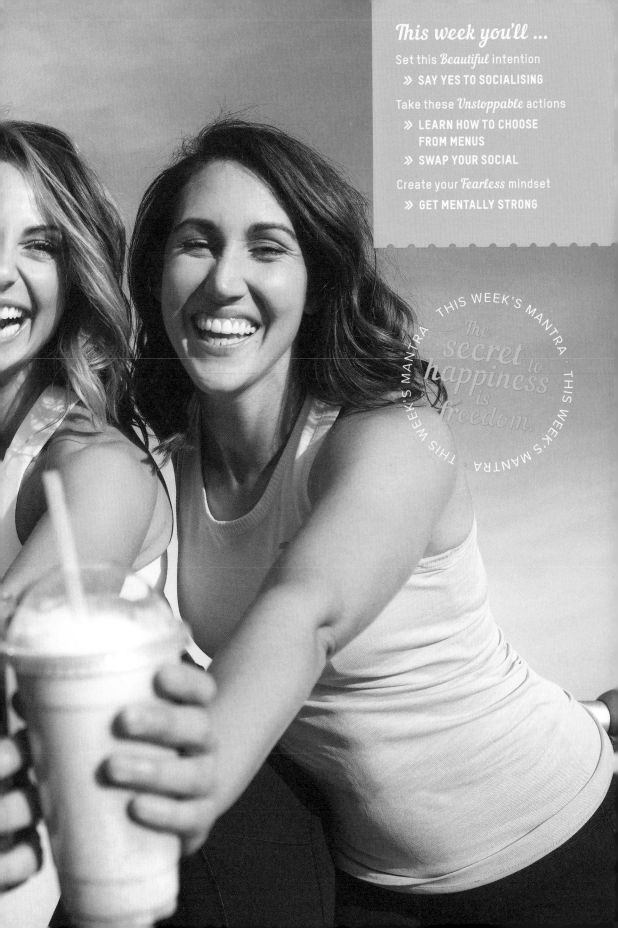

This week you'll ...

Set this *Beautiful* intention
» **SAY YES TO SOCIALISING**

Take these *Unstoppable* actions
» **LEARN HOW TO CHOOSE FROM MENUS**
» **SWAP YOUR SOCIAL**

Create your *Fearless* mindset
» **GET MENTALLY STRONG**

THIS WEEK'S MANTRA · THIS WEEK'S MANTRA · THIS WEEK'S MANTRA · THIS WEEK'S MANTRA ·

The secret to happiness is freedom.

» Say Yes to socialising

This week is all about learning how to stay true to your new healthy standards, wherever you are, without missing out on all the fun. We'll teach you everything from how to choose well from café and restaurant menus to how to navigate a weekend getaway.

We'll also dive into the importance of enjoying 'soul food' from time to time, because life's too short to say 'no thanks' to that gelato on the beach on a hot summer's day!

When you start out on a new health journey, creating some structure is really important – it helps you learn what works for you, set some intentions you can follow through on and figure out how to make the right choices for your body – but now that you're starting to get the hang of all this, it's time to get back to real life.

You've already learned how changing your breakfast can transform your health, that lunch and snack times are opportunities to nourish your body, that you don't have to be a slave to sugar, that you can swap your favourites for healthier options without missing a beat, and that carbohydrates are your friends if you choose the right types. You've also spent a week experimenting with an anti-inflammatory diet and optimising sleep, digestion and hydration. Now it's time to step outside the safety zone of your controlled home/work environments and get a taste of real nutritional freedom.

HERE'S WHAT HAPPENS IF YOU ONLY EVER FOLLOW THE 'RULES'

The first few weeks of a health kick are easy – your motivation is strong and you're loving the results – but three to four weeks in, things can fall apart at the seams.

Typically, people start to fall into one of these two patterns:

#1

Eating healthily at the start of the week, then 'letting go' at the weekend, diving into all the treats circulating on party platters, ordering pancakes at Sunday brunch and guzzling booze because 'you've been good all week'.

#2

Avoiding most social functions and occasions (even dates!) altogether because they're too tempting and you really want to stick to your program.

This week, we challenge you to fall into a third category:

#3

Saying YES to social invitations but at every opportunity turning those outings into nourishing occasions, either for your body or your soul.

A few examples ...

1 You're asked out on a date – say **YES**. Suggest something that fits with your goals – maybe an active date like stand-up paddleboarding, or a walk to a healthy brunch or dinner spot.

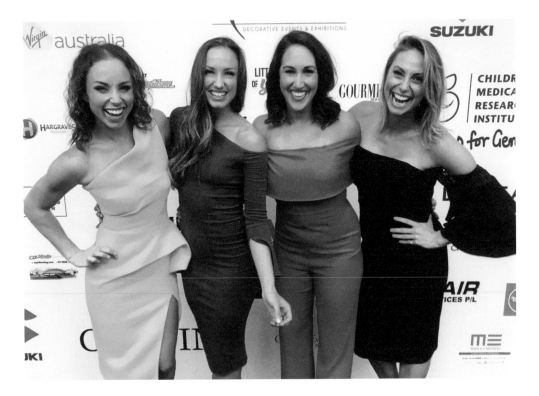

2 Your girlfriends want to go dancing – say **YES**. Stick to a limit of one or two drinks but don't miss out on all the fun. Sip on mineral water in between alcoholic drinks, or grab some sweet, rehydrating coconut water. Worried you won't have enough energy to last all night on the dance floor without booze? This is your chance to use up your coffee allocation – have an espresso, then hit the dance floor with max energy.

3 You're invited to dinner with friends at their choice of restaurant – say **YES**. Check out the restaurant's menu before you go and decide what you'll order before you even get there. The best options will be those that combine a protein source (chicken, fish, etc.) with salad or vegetables. Avoid fried appetisers and sip slowly on one glass of red wine before switching to water. Share a delicious dessert with a friend,

or better yet, the whole table. Oh, and never turn up ravenous!

4 A work function is announced – say **YES**. Make a conscious decision to stick to one or two glasses of alcohol. When it comes to those delicious snacks, reach for fresh options – not fried. You can also try using the rule of five – feel free to indulge in the food being handed around, but stop at your fifth piece.

5 It's a super-special occasion – say **YES**. Whether it's your best friend's birthday, a romantic anniversary, or dinner with your family, special occasions are 'enjoy-the-moment' kind of events. Indulge, let go, eat mindfully and enjoy every single mouthful of that soul food! Do take note of your body and what it's telling you – stop when you're full, sip on water when you need it, and say 'no' to the waiter topping up your wine when you start to feel its effects.

» Learn how to choose from menus

The word of the week is NOT 'guilt' around eating out, it's 'empowerment'. Choosing the healthiest options straight off the menu is one approach to empowered eating. Learning to ask for healthy swaps is another. But figuring out when to throw away the rule book and order what your heart desires – and *not* feel guilty about that – is what we'll address first.

HOW TO DECIDE WHEN TO INDULGE

Sure, it's all about balance: eating healthy foods 80 per cent of the time and treating yourself the other 20 per cent ... but how do you decide when to use that 20 per cent and when to say no?

Think of it this way: you should feel really good about the food you choose to eat, either because it's healthy for you or because it's soul food, meaning you ate it in a shared moment that created a great memory. For example, eating a litre of ice-cream at home in front of the TV by yourself on a week night – that doesn't feel good, does it? But a few scoops of the same ice-cream on a beach in the middle of a hot summer's day, surrounded by friends or family – now *that's* a serve of ice-cream worth having! It's not the food you eat but the context you eat it in, and the attitude you approach it with, that matters. We're human and we don't eat 'nutrients', 'grams', 'calories' and 'portions', we eat meals shared with family, lunches that provide respite from a busy work day, treats with our friends or kids on weekends, and glasses of wine shared over easy conversation with the person we love at the end of a big week.

Eat mindfully. Let some meals nourish your body and others nourish your soul.

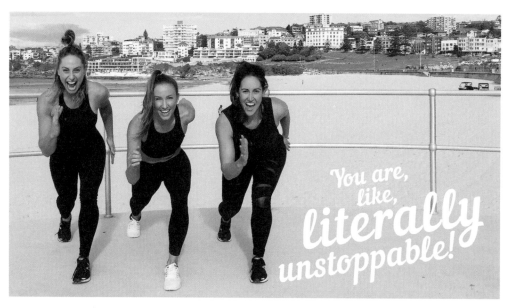

You are, like, *literally* unstoppable!

HEALTHY ORDERING

Here's a quick guide to what to order and avoid with some of the most common cuisines.

VIETNAMESE
ORDER rice paper rolls, salads and pho soup
AVOID deep-fried options, spring rolls and creamy sauces

JAPANESE
ORDER brown rice sushi, sashimi, grilled meats, miso soup, seaweed, salads, edamame and steamed dumplings
AVOID anything with 'tempura', 'fried' or 'teriyaki' in the title, white rice (most places use sugar to make it sticky), thick miso sauces, and if you're avoiding gluten, soy sauce

SPANISH
ORDER tapas made from grilled lamb, calamari and fish, grilled veggies and a splash of Spanish red wine
AVOID fried potatoes, Spanish breads, aioli, and definitely the churros!

MEXICAN
ORDER traditional Mexican meals packed with vegetables or salad, beans and rice, corn tortillas and spicy chilli or salsa, and feel free to order the guacamole on the side
AVOID the corn chips, wheat tortillas and sugary cocktails (just ask them to leave the sugar or syrup out), and the sour cream too

NEW-STYLE FISH 'N' CHIPS
ORDER grilled fish with salad or veggies and maybe even a side of rice instead (if your fish 'n' chips shop sells it)
AVOID deep-fried and battered fish, potato scallops and hot chips

INDIAN
ORDER grilled meats and vegetables, panak peneer (grilled spinach and cottage cheese), cucumber raita, dahl and tomato-based dishes, ideally with the sauce on the side
AVOID naan breads, butter chicken, creamy curries and deep-fried entrees

YOUR LOCAL PUB OR FAVOURITE AUSSIE RESTAURANT
ORDER a basic protein (meat, chicken, fish) with vegetables or salad and any sauces on the side, plus roast potato or sweet potato and a glass of wine
AVOID hot chips, creamy sauces, crumbed or fried foods, cheeses and crisps

YOUR FAVOURITE CAFÉ
ORDER eggs and frittatas, salad greens or leaves, any vegetables like mushrooms or asparagus, savoury fruits like tomato or avocado, sourdough or rye toast, smoked salmon, occasionally bacon (if you know it comes from a good-quality source), porridge or muesli with no added honey or syrup (or get it on the side), fresh fruit and plain yoghurt, whole milk or nut milk, fresh vegetable juices
AVOID white bread, deep-fried fritters, banana bread, muffins and baked goods, fruit juices, breakfast sausages, granolas, pancakes, waffles and doughnuts

BURGER BAR
ORDER your choice of burger with salad and pickles – with or without the bun!
AVOID fries, and too much cheese

PIZZA
ORDER thin-crust pizza of your choice, with just a quarter to half the regular amount of cheese, and extra vegetables and a side salad
AVOID deep-pan pizzas, triple-cheese pizzas, garlic breads

ITALIAN
ORDER minestrone soup, salad, bruschetta, pastas with red sauce (and ask for extra veggies/protein and less actual pasta), fresh fish, antipasto
AVOID creamy sauces, garlic breads, cheese-loaded pizzas, heavy desserts

MIDDLE EASTERN
ORDER hummus and babaganoush, pita bread, tabouleh, greens, baked eggs and animal proteins, legumes
AVOID Gyro sandwiches, Turkish coffee, fried potatoes, deep-fried falafel or kibbeh

THAI
ORDER any protein- and vegetable-packed dish you like, with *all* sauces on the side
AVOID fried and battered foods

CHINESE
ORDER Chinese broccoli, stir-fried mixed vegetables, chicken with cashew nuts, steamed dumplings
AVOID deep-fried and battered options, and sweet/salty sauces

HOW TO CONFIDENTLY ASK FOR SWAPS

It can initially be a bit confronting asking for variations on what's on the menu at a restaurant or café, but the more you do it, the more confident you become and the easier it is to eat the way you really want to. Be clear and confident, not embarrassed. You're the customer, and asking for a menu modification is totally acceptable. If you feel embarrassed asking for swaps in front of friends, you can always call the restaurant ahead of your visit and explain your dietary needs to them, so they're aware and prepared.

Be flexible, and keep changes simple. Asking for four or five changes to your meal might get a little too much, but small tweaks are much more likely to be accepted easily by both the wait staff and your friends. Switch a side of fries to a side salad, ask for your pizza without the cheese, request gluten-free bread, or switch the bacon for avocado, sure, but don't overcomplicate things by asking for the triple-cheese pasta with seafood, minus the cheese, with gluten-free pasta, using chicken instead of seafood and with sauce on the side.

And tell the truth. If you're experimenting with going grain free, don't lie and say you have a gluten allergy. Just be honest, otherwise things can get awkward fast.

HEALTHIEST ALCOHOL OPTIONS

It's so easy to underestimate liquid calories, but they sure do add up. Avoid soft drinks, pre-made mixers, anything frozen, anything creamy, anything made with an energy drink, and shots. Check out this list of the healthiest drinks you can order at the bar:

Red or white wine 1 serve (150 ml) has around 100–150 calories and minimal

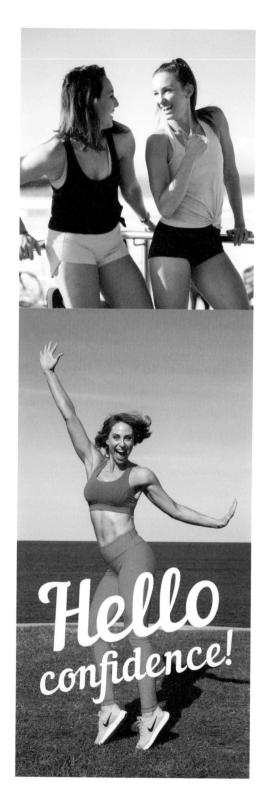

Hello confidence!

sugar. Red wine is our pick, due to all the antioxidants.

Vodka with soda water and fresh lime 1 serve contains just over 100 calories and the lime reduces the glycaemic index (GI) of the drink, so your blood sugars rise more slowly and won't 'crash' afterwards.

Light beer Be aware that this choice contains gluten and a few other ingredients that can cause bloating, but it's not a bad option if you stop at one.

Bloody Mary A bloody Mary is light on calories and packed with antioxidants, the spices and peppers give your metabolism a little boost, and the celery adds freshness and fibre. This drink fills you up, so you're less likely to crave a second drink.

Margaritas We're not talking the frozen, pre-mixed kind of margarita, and you've got to ask the bartender not to use sugar syrup or agave, just straight up tequila, Cointreau and fresh lime juice. Tequila is one of the only alcohols that acts as a mood booster, rather than a depressant.

'Dry' cocktails Ask the bartender for a dry cocktail with no added sugar. He's sure to know a few tricks of the trade to help you out.

Quality champagne Sparkles are lighter on calories than wine, at about 90 calories per serve, but they do have a bit more sugar.

Gin & tonic Hold the tonic! People often assume that because it's called 'tonic *water*' this is a good choice, but tonic water actually has as much sugar as a can of cola. Have your gin with soda water instead.

HEALTHIEST COFFEE ORDERS
Note: these are based on using whole-fat milk or substitutes, because our philosophy is always to eat the food that's least processed.

Espresso or long black These literally only contain a few calories each.

Piccolo latte or Americano These contain less than 50 calories.

Other coffee orders are okay in moderation, but keep in mind that they will all have more than 150 calories per cup, with items like a large latte or mocha coming in at 300–400 calories.

TREAT ... OR TRICK?
Are these seemingly healthy treats playing tricks with your body? Scan this list to make sure your social snacking habits aren't betraying you!

Skinny latte Compared to whole milk, skim milk is typically higher in sugar, less satiating and can mess with your appetite hormones, as it's not a 'complete' food. So consider skipping that skinny latte and reaching for a long black with a generous splash of organic full-cream milk instead. When it comes to cappuccinos, here's a heads-up: that delish choc topping is pretty much all sugar and no cocoa.

Some dark chocolate brands We love dark chocolate and it has incredible health benefits, BUT ... there are healthy, low-sugar brands and then there are others that come loaded with as much sugar and often more fat than their milk chocolate cousins. Make sure you don't stop at the claims of '70% cocoa'; check the nutritional label too, and look for options with less than 10 g of sugar per 100 g.

Trail mix Yep, nuts are healthy, but moreish trail mixes often come with sugary dried fruit and a lashing of unhealthy vegetable oils, too. You're better off buying raw or activated nuts, coconut flakes and some healthy dried fruits, like goji berries or freeze-dried blueberries, and making your own mix.

Mocktails Yep, saying no to alcohol is great, but ordering mocktails to fill the gap can be a calorie-laden mistake, as they're often full of fruit juices and syrups. The exception is a Virgin Mary ... order up!

Sushi train Sushi seems like a good choice, and in moderation it can be, but most sushi trains use sugar to make their rice sticky, plus they serve sauces and mayonnaise full of sugar and unhealthy fats. Instead of filling up on roll after starchy roll, just choose the safer menu items: edamame beans, sashimi, seaweed salad and a small serve of your favourite sushi roll to make sure you feel satisfied.

'No added sugar' carob Carob still has a lot of sugar in it, without adding a thing. This doesn't mean it's unhealthy, it just means you need to watch your portions.

Sugar-free and zero-calorie soda Drinking diet soft drinks can not only contribute to the development of type 2 diabetes, it confuses your appetite hormones and has been proven to make most people put on weight in the long-term. Most are loaded with toxic chemicals, too – no thanks!

Bircher muesli Sure, soaking your oats overnight is the healthiest way to prepare them, but if you're getting the store- or café-bought kind, 99 per cent of the time they're soaked in apple juice and have honey and raisins added. That equals one big sugar fest. And don't even think about ordering that Acai bowl with a sprinkling of granola – it's sugar central! Prep your own grains like a true BUF Girl. ☺

Protein bars A lot of protein bars are loaded with chemicals, fake sugars, synthetic vitamins, cheap protein powders and preservatives. Look for brands with minimal ingredients and no nasty artificial sugars. Even the 'good' choices tend to be high on calories, so use sweet protein bars as a treat, not something you eat every single time you hit the gym, and certainly not in place of real food.

Honey and agave syrup These two have their health benefits, but they're also both very high in fructose and have a similar impact on blood glucose levels as regular, refined sugar, so go easy on your portion sizes. Our pick of the two is raw honey, or swap it for fructose-free maple or rice malt syrups.

SOCIAL HABITS Q&A

Changing your social habits can be hard to do, so here are the questions and concerns the BUF Girls community bring up most often on this topic.

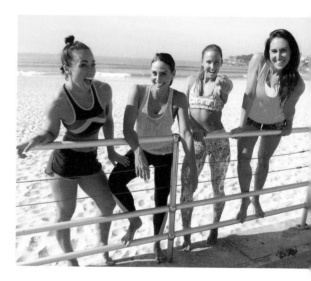

I have the best of intentions, but then suddenly I'm at an event, snacking on naughty finger food. What are the best options?
Steer clear of fried foods and carbohydrate-dense options. Reach for olives, nuts, grilled protein or veggie skewers, smoked salmon on crisp-bread, fruit, hummus, ceviche, rice paper rolls and sushi. Have one or two drinks with lots of water or sparkling water in between.

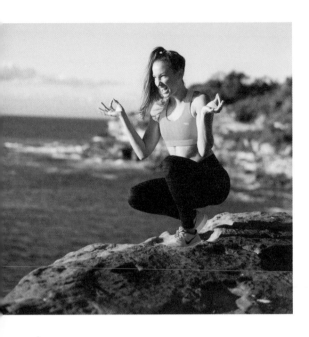

In the meantime, either gently suggest a different kind of catch-up (walk, movies, massage, health-conscious restaurant, picnic in the great outdoors, a girls' movie night in), or accept the bar invite and just have one drink you sip on slowly, then order mineral water with fresh mint and lime, or a Virgin Mary.

Enjoy catching up with your friend with a clear mind, while still in an environment she feels comfortable and happy in. Don't push your choices on her, either. Just because you're on a get-healthy, feel-fabulous mission doesn't mean she has to be!

I've been asked out on a date at a trendy bar and I'd love to go, but it's no-booze week ... help!
First of all, say **YES** to that date. Go, enjoy a glass of wine or two but stop there and not just because you're midway through your program – you definitely want to keep your wits about you on a first date! Flushed and flirty after a nice glass of wine is perfect, but slurring and sleepy? Not so hot.

I have one friend in particular who only wants to catch up with me over a few (or many) glasses of alcohol. How can I stop getting sucked into boozy nights out?
Some friends will naturally be more supportive than others when it comes to your health endeavours, but peer pressure is no reason to cave in. You can only be responsible for your own actions and your good friends will gradually accept your decision.

I'm heading overseas on a holiday. Do I just forget healthy eating and start over when I get home?
Eating healthy food should be starting to become something you *want* to do, not just something you feel obliged to do. Treat your overseas holiday as you would your weekends at home, indulging in and enjoying healthy, nourishing and yummy foods, having the occasional treat, enjoying a cheeky wine but stopping at one or two, sampling the local delicacies but not gorging. It's all about balance.

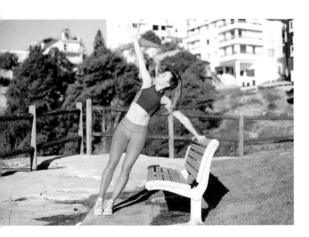

» Swap your social

This week's unstoppable fitness action is to swap one of your usual social outings for a more active 'fit date' and see whether it isn't just as much fun as your usual routine – maybe even more so!

Here are our date ideas for every kind of partner in crime (friend, date, family member) ...

The outdoorsy type Take a big long walk in the great outdoors, or maybe even spend a whole day going walkabout. This is one of our favourite things to do: pack a backpack with a few essentials like food, water, a swimsuit, a towel and a good book, then just walk from one place to the other, adventuring all day long! Check out wildwalks.com for ideas.

The sports lover Book a tennis court and have a hit, pick up a football or basketball and head to a local park or court, nab your brother's skateboard and learn how to ride it, or book a surfing lesson.

The big kid Remember playing laser tag or skirmish as a kid? They're both just as great as an adult! Or you and your friend could download the app Zombies Run onto your phones and start playing. Check it out at zombiesrungame.com.

The socialite Book a group adventure – a cycling tour through a local wine region, a kayak tour out on the ocean, a dance class or a picnic in the park with all your girlfriends, followed by a big walk and gossip session.

The gym junkie Google the workouts of one of your favourite celebrities or athletes, print it out then meet at the gym and do it with your friend. Alternatively, look up a group class neither of you have tried before and book your spots. Follow the sweat sesh with a brunch date.

The beach addict Find a beach you have to walk through a bit of bush to get to, then pack a day bag and go for it. There are heaps of these gems sprinkled through national parks around Australia.

The adrenaline junkie Anything that gives a thrill will do nicely. From rock climbing and abseiling to canyoning, high ropes, a cross-country bike tour, water skiing or wakeboarding, snorkelling or diving, or even hitting up a water park.

The Rocky wannabe Book a boxing class you can do together and hit out all your stress from the week.

The escape artist If all your friend/partner talks about are holidays, day trips, weekends away and escaping the rat race, book a weekender and go exploring on foot.

The night owl Swap the nightclub for a dark spin studio with epic tunes.

Swap, don't stop!

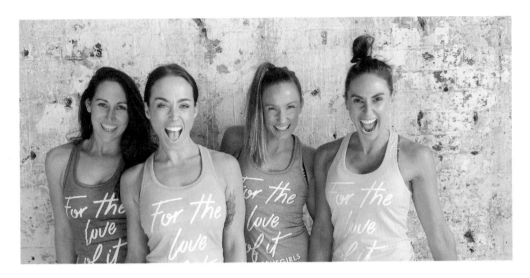

THIS WEEK'S (F)EARLESS MINDSET
» Get mentally strong

It takes commitment to take your healthy lifestyle out of the home and into your social zone, but it's Week Five and you've come a long way. This week's fearless mindset intention is to build a little mental resilience.

Check out our ideas to get mentally strong – think of it as flexing and toning your mind muscle ...

FIVE TIPS TO GET MENTALLY STRONG

1. Learn to let things go
Nobody is perfect, yet so many of us hold lofty standards for ourselves, and struggle in the face of failure.

News flash: everybody fails! In fact, failure can be a really good thing, it helps you to learn and grow. Don't allow yourself to worry endlessly about that one session you missed, or the piece of chocolate cake you ate. Without failures there would be no lessons learned, or new heights reached.

One of our favourite BUF mantras is to use guilt as a guide for what to do better next time, rather than as a weapon against yourself – and we really believe in putting that into practice. If you allow yourself to be pulled down by slip-ups and wrong turns, you will never be able to move forward. So give yourself a break and focus on the lessons you're learning and the person you're becoming as you go through this journey.

2. Focus on the present
Humans find it very hard to stay in the present moment. We get caught up in thoughts of what happened yesterday, or what may happen tomorrow, while the present moment – the only thing we really have control over – passes us by.

A simple way to draw your attention to the present is to use cue words and affirmations, for example 'breathe' or 'pause and ground yourself'.

3. Stay positive and productive

You don't have to be all smiles when you're not feeling great, however it can be helpful to replace negative thinking with energising thoughts.

A simple example of this might be when you're training and feel the session is too hard for you. Rather than telling yourself, 'I can't do this', or, 'I'm so bad at push-ups/burpees/etc.', simply replace that thought with, 'I am strong', 'I am athletic', or 'I love how my body feels when it moves'.

If you honestly can't complete something, don't beat yourself up about it. Use the experience to set yourself a new goal; for example, 'I'm going to practise every day so that I'm able to complete 10 push-ups on my toes by the end of the year'.

It's about continually catching your thoughts and rewiring them so they're helpful and moving you forward, rather than acting like an anchor.

4. Use rituals and visuals

Human beings are creatures of habit, and the better the habits you create for yourself, the better your results will be.

Successful athletes have clear rituals or cues to help them perform better, like mantras (I am an athlete! I feel strong! I perform best when the going gets tough!), visuals (imagining they're chasing down a competitor) and distraction techniques (like repeating the alphabet, or singing their favourite song in their heads and focusing on staying in time with the rhythm).

It takes 21 days to set a new habit, and it all begins with the little actions you take daily, so start now! You might begin with something as simple as replacing your evening chocolate treat with a herbal tea, getting up 30 minutes earlier to exercise, or picking a song to play that gets you in the mood for your workout each day. Whatever you choose to focus on, make sure each ritual energises you and encourages a positive state of mind.

5. Learn to love the journey more than the destination

It is so vital that you enjoy the path you're on and acknowledge that it's not all about getting a particular result. The journey itself can be the reward. For example, you may think, 'I'll be happy when the scale says 60 kg', or, 'I'll be happy when I can fit into that dress', but all you can control is the moment you find yourself in right now, so keep moving towards your goal but focus on the little wins you're having right here, today. You just chose a healthy salad over a burger – well done! You really enjoyed learning to make BUF bliss balls, woo-hoo!

There's no point dwelling on thoughts of what 'might be' some day. Make fitness and healthy eating an integral and exciting part of your life, not a means to an end.

THE POWER OF PRESENCE

This week, try being deeply present when you spend time with your friends, family or partner. Put your phone away and listen deeply. Watch their facial expressions, feel their energy – just be truly present with them in each moment.

Observing someone can be a powerful gift, but it is also good for you, grounding you in the moment and taking you out of your own head and into someone else's heart.

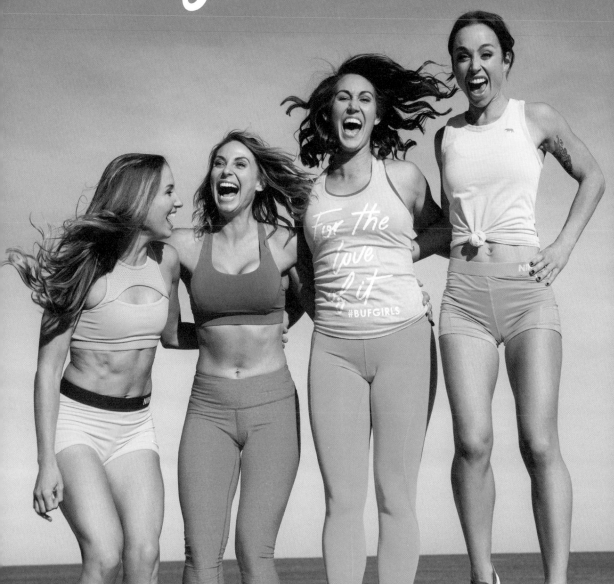

TOP TIPS 'n' TAKEAWAYS

» The secret to happiness is freedom, so always remember that the point of using a structured food plan is not to need a structured food plan ever again!

» Don't be afraid to say YES to social invites – simply put a little thought into the food and drink choices you make when out and about so you can stay healthy and wake up feeling amazing the next day.

» If you're heading out on the town, do a quick scan of our healthiest cuisines and alcoholic drinks lists and steer your night in the right direction.

» If in doubt, a protein source (without the sauce) and a serve of green vegetables or salad is spot-on. Feel free to add the roast potatoes, but ditch the fried ones. ☺

» Take a friend or partner out for a 'fit date' this week.

» Mental muscles are as important as physical ones, if not more, so make sure you flex them!

WEEK FIVE
MEAL PLAN

	Breakfast	*Lunch*	*Dinner*
MONDAY	Carrot Cake Oats PAGE 105	Crispy Chicken Salad PAGE 150	Cashew Butter Stir-fry PAGE 186
TUESDAY	Coco Quinoa Bowl PAGE 108	Mushroom and Tuna Bake PAGE 156	Hearty Bolognese with Zucchini 'Pasta' PAGE 194
WEDNESDAY	Breakfast Tortilla PAGE 104	Pho Bowl PAGE 162	Pan-fried Steak with Sautéed Greens PAGE 210
THURSDAY	Bubble and Squeak PAGE 104	Brown Rice Poke Bowl PAGE 140	Chicken Burgers with Sweet Potato Chips PAGE 188
FRIDAY	Very Vegetable Fritters PAGE 125	Cheeseburger with Carrot Fries PAGE 144	Sweet Potato Gnocchi PAGE 222

Snack options

» HEALTHY STRAWBERRY CRUMBLE (PAGE 238)
» FRENCH ONION DIP (PAGE 247)
» FUDGY BEAN BROWNIES (PAGE 236)
» VANILLA CRUSH (PAGE 245)

Live a BUF
Life

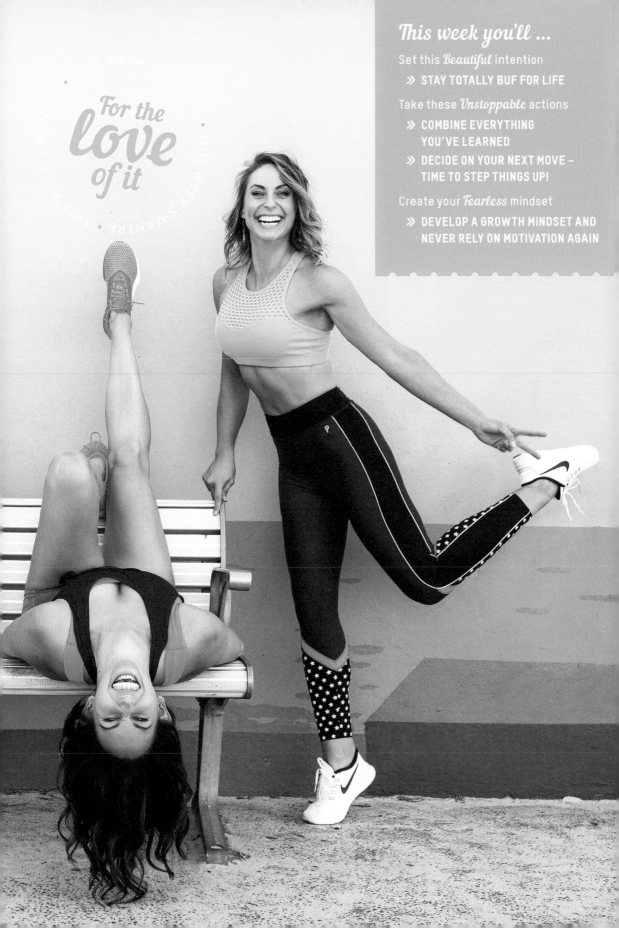

For the
love
of it

This week you'll ...

Set this *Beautiful* intention

» **STAY TOTALLY BUF FOR LIFE**

Take these *Unstoppable* actions

» **COMBINE EVERYTHING YOU'VE LEARNED**

» **DECIDE ON YOUR NEXT MOVE – TIME TO STEP THINGS UP!**

Create your *Fearless* mindset

» **DEVELOP A GROWTH MINDSET AND NEVER RELY ON MOTIVATION AGAIN**

» Stay totally BUF for life

It's time to put every skill you've learned over the past five weeks together for one clean-eating, action-packed week – we're coming home strong!

This week is all about embracing and enjoying your new lifestyle, and setting you up to feel forever (B)eautiful, inside and out, (U)nstoppable with the support of an amazing tribe of women around you, and (F)earless in the pursuit of whatever goals you have.

Putting it all together means this week you'll be:

1   eating protein, healthy fat and fibre-packed foods for breakfast

2   avoiding the refined sugar rollercoaster

3   reaching for the healthiest version of the food you're craving

4   consciously choosing fibre-rich wholegrains over refined carbohydrates

5   ditching processed and packaged snacks, as well as unhealthy trans fats

6   including anti-inflammatory foods

7   not relying on caffeine to get through your day

8   using the 1–2 rule for alcohol consumption

9   potentially using some basic supplements to boost results, like a good-quality fish oil and some magnesium oil before bed, or some BUF Girls' protein powder

10 saying yes to socialising and practising making healthy menu choices

That's ten incredible habits you've nailed in five short weeks. Well done!

Hopefully by now you're starting to really enjoy eating fresher, healthier food, upgrading your understanding of how the body works and moving your body for the love of it.

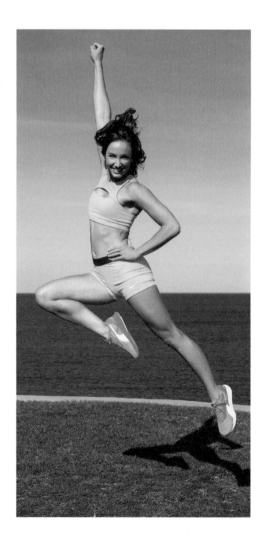

» Combine everything you've learned

In a world where everyone is addicted to the quick fix, we're making a stand for consistency because healthy, lasting change certainly doesn't happen overnight. However, if you can make eating fresh food and regularly moving your body a part of who you are, the results can truly last a lifetime. The healthiest, fittest people we know regard good eating and exercise as a gift rather than a chore.

Take a moment to reflect on and feel grateful for how far you've come. Even if you feel you still have a lot further to go, that's totally okay because you have the rest of your life to keep building on your new skills. Keep reminding yourself to let go of your need for short-term results and set some clear intentions for the kind of healthy life you want to live, then commit to taking small actions daily that improve things, one workout, meal or meditation at a time.

Here's a cheat list to help you stay on track this week, and every week from here on in …

Meal mantras

We love using powerful, meaningful words to drive our breakfast, lunch and dinner choices. Simply bring the word relating to each meal to the front of your mind before you decide what to eat, and we promise you'll be more inclined to go for the good stuff!

BREAKFAST = ENERGY (what will you eat that will set you up for a great day?)

LUNCH = FUEL (what lunch choice will keep you powering through the afternoon?)

DINNER = NOURISH (how well can you nourish your body after a big day?)

Eat more wholefoods and minimise processed foods

Fresh plant- and animal-based foods in as close to their natural state as possible will help keep your metabolism functioning at its best. Processed foods provide much less nourishment and can contribute to weight gain and metabolic disease.

Keep your liver clean

Your liver is a powerhouse when it comes to burning fat. Help this super-efficient organ do its job by minimising alcohol (use the 1–2 principle), refined carbohydrates, sugar and trans fats.

Eat protein at breakfast

The protein breakfast is your biggest weapon when it comes to defending yourself against the biscuit or lolly jar. Not only will making sure you get some protein into your first meal of the day have you burning fat from the outset, it will also keep your blood sugar levels under control and prevent cravings. The cherry on top? You'll also feel more focused throughout the morning and determined to get through your to-do list, as protein fires up your brain!

Avoid sugar

Excessive sugar consumption not only encourages your body to store fat and puts your health at risk, it also ages your skin. Practise saying no to the obvious culprits but also avoid hidden sources, like those found in processed foods, sauces, starches and takeaways.

Pay attention to nutrients, not calories

Before you sit down to meals, say to yourself, 'I am a healthy person', and choose what to eat from that place. A focus on how much good stuff you can get in, rather than how much you have to cut out, feels more flexible, fun and achievable.

Prioritise sleep

Sleep deprivation will make you hungry, moody, anxious, unmotivated and, in the long run, overweight and unwell. Prioritise sleep, and if you find you're restless at night time, try using a magnesium supplement or oil to nod off.

Stay hydrated

Just 2 per cent dehydration can have a huge effect on your energy levels, appetite hormones and physical performance. Drink up to live it up!

Don't think 'diet', think 'life culture'

Diets are so last century. Shift the whole way you're thinking by focusing on creating an incredible, active, healthy, happy culture for your life instead. Take little actions every day that fuel the lifestyle you've chosen, and focus on enjoying the journey, not striving for a final destination.

MAINTENANCE MODE – SAY NO TO THE YO-YO!

A lot of women don't realise that maintaining their ideal body shape long-term takes an entirely different skill set to losing weight in the first place. Understanding how to shift gears is incredibly important if you don't want to turn into a human yo-yo, losing and gaining weight over and over again.

Here's a rundown on what the 'leaning out' and 'maintenance' phases are all about:

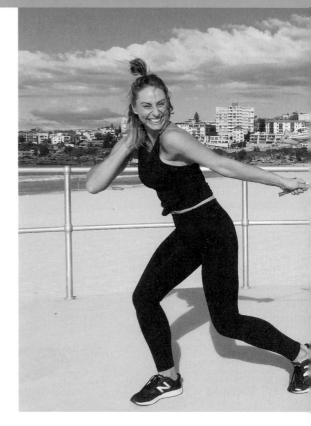

LEANING OUT is for learning new skills, practising self-control, eating by the book, being aware of portions and restricting temptation foods to reset your body and metabolism, as well as shaking things up with a fitness push.

MAINTENANCE is more about moderation, consistency and balance, as well as making an ongoing commitment to your health goals and really paying attention to what works for you and your body. It's about staying curious: continuing to learn, and experimenting with what makes your body feel good. It's also very important to take a relaxed but mindful approach to both your nutrition and fitness as you move into this phase, which is all about setting yourself up for life.

There are a few more things to keep in mind as you step into this new phase, where body acceptance and slowing down are just as important as all that dedication and consistency you have demonstrated in getting BUF.

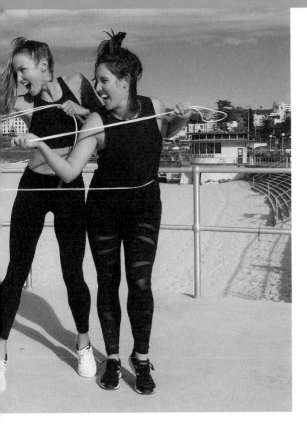

Keep moving

Your body was made to move, so stay focused on creating that movement culture for you and your family. The more time you spend seated, the harder it is for your body to stay healthy and fit, so aim for 30–60 minutes of movement every day, even if it's just a walk in the sunshine, or a BUF workout in your lounge room (join us online at bufgirls.com!).

Be confident

It's okay to say 'no thanks' when family and friends try to push that second piece of cake, or third glass of wine, into your hand. Set yourself a little challenge to stand up for your health goals and you may even score some new skills in assertiveness and self-belief while you're at it. Good friends will admire your strength, and as for family, well, they'll love you no matter what.

Be prepared

You have to prepare if you want to win, so if you know you're going to a social gathering where there will be nothing nutritious for you to eat, take some emergency rations, or better yet, offer to bring a plate to share.

Sip, don't gulp

We're talking alcohol here! Sip on one or two delicious glasses of red wine all evening, or allow yourself a few cocktails, but then stop and switch to sparkling water with some fresh lime and mint thrown in for good measure. You'll still look like you're in on the fun but will be refreshing your body and clearing your mind.

Eat consistently

There's no set number of times you 'should' eat per day, but it can be helpful to never quite get to the point of being desperate for whatever comes your way. If you starve yourself during the day so you've 'got room' for all the treats on offer at dinner, you're almost guaranteed to overindulge. Eat regularly, when you feel hungry but not ravenous, and remember to eat protein or a small portion of good fats at every meal to keep you satisfied and avoid nasty cravings.

Resolution *now*

You don't have to wait until another New Year's Day rocks around to make a resolution. We love to set ourselves mini goals regularly, and a really fun way to do this is to grab yourself an old-school wall calendar and set yourself a new goal each month, which you commit to doing every day until you turn to a fresh page. Cross each day off as you complete your mini resolution and see if you can get to the end of the month without missing a single day.

Refined sugar is devilish

Skipping out on sugary desserts and refined carbohydrates is a great idea most of the time, as they can stress your body out. Simply having this awareness around sweet foods will steer you towards healthier choices and then, when you do indulge, you can really enjoy every devilishly good mouthful.

Naughty can be nice
A treat here and there will not have a negative impact on your health if you're consistent with eating well and moving your body most of the time, so don't be too hard on yourself if you slip up – just wake up the next day and get back on track with your healthy eating and exercise plan. It's all about consistency.

Make your workouts social
Fitness isn't just about getting fit; it's a chance to catch up with a great girlfriend, connect with your partner, meet new people or bond with your kids. Getting active with people creates a deeper kind of bond, one that's worth making time for.

Recovery is where the magic happens
Tough training is great, so long as you help your body recover from it, because that recovery time is where the magic happens. It's when you go for a walk, or do some yoga the day after a hard workout, that your body has a chance to recover, tone up and slim down. Listen to your body and be okay with swapping a tough circuit or run for a good walk or stretch when you feel you need it.

You are capable of amazing things!

Beauty begins within
The most beautiful girls are the happy, kind and caring girls, so remember not to focus too much on how you look but rather on how you live and act towards others.

Find out what you enjoy …
And do more of it. If you don't like running, you don't need to force yourself to do it. Everyone's physiology is different, so find what is fun for you and do more of it to maintain a positive association with fitness.

KEEP YOUR KITCHEN STOCKED WITH THESE

Now that you're all schooled up on nutrition and what works for you, it's time to take a look at our top everyday superfoods. Keep these in your kitchen so you always have nutrient-dense options on hand.

Salmon, mackerel and sardines Salmon, mackerel and sardines are high in protein and *super*-high in healthy, essential fats. The canned versions are great little convenience options.

Berries Berries are low in sugar but high in fibre, as well as high in the antioxidants that fight free radicals, preventing the cell damage that leads to disease and ageing. Raspberries contain a unique antioxidant that can improve the brain's sensitivity to leptin, making you feel less hungry, while blueberries help you focus at work.

Eggs Organic and free-range eggs are a great source of protein, folate, vitamin B_{12}, phosphorus and selenium, while being low in salt. Eat the yolk and the white for maximum benefits.

Leafy greens Greens such as spinach, kale, chard and lettuce are low in calories and carbohydrates and high in phytonutrients, which protect you from environmental stressors and boost immunity.

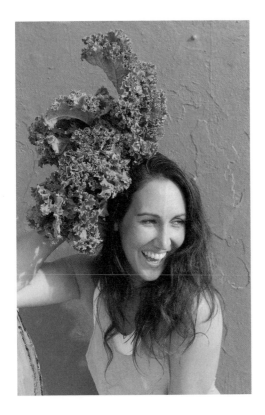

it contains. Green tea also helps to regulate blood glucose levels (thus stabilising insulin response) and inhibits the process of carbohydrates being stored as fat – it helps you burn that energy instead! The recommended dose is 2–3 big mugs of hot or chilled tea. Don't add sugar or other sweeteners.

Nuts Nuts are high in antioxidants, protein, fibre and healthy fats, and research shows the hormone leptin (satiety hormone) has been found to be higher in people who eat nuts daily.

Avocados Avocados are high in good fats, helping to lower bad cholesterol and reduce inflammation. They also help you lose fat by improving insulin sensitivity.

Lemon, lime and grapefruit Eat these health-giving fruits from the citrus family first thing in the morning for a metabolic boost, squeeze them over your meals to lower the overall glycaemic index, enjoy them as a healthy snack, or squeeze them into your water. They're some of the healthiest little pockets of goodness around!

A DAY ON OUR PLATES

We know you just can't resist a peek at what your trainers like to nosh on, so we've included details on the next couple of pages. ☺ It's also worth taking note of just how different each of our days look. There are so many different ways to create a healthy life!

Cruciferous vegetables Cruciferous vegetables such as cauliflower, broccoli, bok choy, kale, asparagus and cabbage are high in fibre and contain phytonutrients that help oestrogen metabolism. This means they're really great for helping you lean down in the legs and hip area.

Chicken Free-range chicken contains the perfect ratio of omega 3 to omega 6 fats. It's also a great source of bio-available protein, which means it's easier to digest. The recommended amount is 100 g uncooked per serving (double that for men), containing about 25 g of protein.

Green tea Green tea is a natural source of caffeine, increasing your metabolic rate and enhancing your training capacity. The good thing is that green tea won't give you a racing heart and anxiety, as coffee often does, thanks to the particular antioxidants

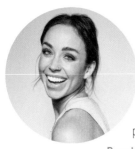

Alicia

When I wake up A big glass of water, then a piccolo.

Breakfast I try to change what I have for breakfast day to day. Some days it will be an omelette with lots of greens such as kale and zucchini, plus goat's feta on top, or avocado on a slice of good-quality bread, or a smoothie with a coconut-water base, cucumber, protein powder, spinach, frozen berries and a little scoop of almond butter. Variety is key!

Lunch Lunch is nearly always a homemade, or healthy café salad with some kind of protein (smoked salmon, chicken), plus sweet potato or pumpkin and a green base. I'm obsessed with miso, hummus and chilli to add flavour and some excitement to my salads. If I'm really organised I'll bake up a heap of roast veggies to add to homemade salads, too.

Dinner I'm not the greatest chef, so unless someone's cooking for me, it's always something super-simple and generally fairly light, as I tend to eat bigger meals at breakfast and lunch. I like baking chicken, salmon or white fish with herbs and spices (it's hard to ruin things too much in the oven), and greens steamed in a bamboo basket with a cube of ginger. I'm also good with stir-fries - a little coconut oil, mixed veggies, a protein source and flash-fry it all up!

Dessert I have a serious sweet tooth! I love carob chocolate and also slightly sweet homemade popcorn (air popped and drizzled with a bit of honey or maple syrup).

Snacks I love bananas and apples, nuts, or good old boiled eggs with some pepper.

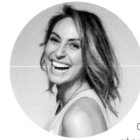

Cassey

When I wake up I love water with a touch of apple cider vinegar to kick-start my metabolism and hydrate my body after a sleep.

Breakfast In winter I like to have porridge cooked in coconut milk, with berries, half a banana, cinnamon and a tablespoon of nut butter. In summer I often have a green smoothie made with BUF Girls' protein powder, fresh spinach, nut butter, a quarter avocado, half a banana, plus coconut milk or coconut water.

Lunch If I'm at home I usually make a big omelette jam-packed with as many veggies as I can, then top it all off with feta and cayenne pepper. If on the run I'll grab a green breakfast bowl or avocado on toast. I love to have breakfast foods for lunch!

Dinner My go-to meal is salmon with sautéed greens (see recipe page 208). So easy to make, and packed with all the goodness I need.

Dessert Chamomile tea with a pinch of stevia powder and some coconut milk, and a few squares of 90% dark chocolate on the side.

Snacks Peanut butter on an apple slice (see recipe page 242).

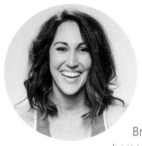

Sian

When I wake up A big mug of peppermint tea

Breakfast If I'm at home I'll have a breakfast bowl (see recipe page 124). Packing loads of nutrient-dense foods into my day is important for my energy levels, which is why I love to get a good head start with a breakfast that's bursting at the seams with good-quality wholefoods. If I'm on the run, I'll have a slice of homemade asparagus, rocket and tomato quiche with an almond meal base. This is the easiest thing for me to whip up at the start of the week and eat on the go if I'm busy.

Lunch I always make up a big salad at the start of the week and keep it in the fridge. One of my favourites is baby spinach, cannellini beans, avocado, cherry tomatoes, red onion and goat's cheese topped with a homemade seeded mustard dressing. I then simply throw some in a container with whatever leftover meat I've got in the fridge from the night before, and there's a perfect lunch for the office.

Dinner My go-to is oven-baked salmon parcels with lemon, chilli and dill, served with a side of sweet potato chips and steamed broccolini. I prefer to eat white meat or fish for dinner to avoid having a heavy meal still sitting in my belly when I head to bed.

Dessert If I have dessert then it's definitely chocolate! I'm a big fan of any dark chocolate with sea salt in it.

Snacks Natural yoghurt mixed with chocolate protein powder topped with strawberries, almonds and coconut chips.

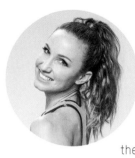

Libby

When I wake up A big glass of warm water with a squeeze of lemon, then either herbal tea or, on big mornings, a Bulletproof® coffee.

Breakfast I'm a late-morning breakfast eater. I usually train others and myself first, so when I do get to it, breakfast is my favourite and biggest meal of the day, always packed with protein. I'll have either a few eggs with veggies or salad and a piece of sourdough, or some Greek or sheep's milk yoghurt with Nutty Granola (see recipe page 116) and a handful of berries.

Lunch Salad with some kind of protein, plus avocado and a starch like quinoa, sweet potato, pumpkin or rice.

Dinner My husband and I are both busy, so on a Sunday I'll often prep a big batch of one of the BUF salads and also the Veggie or Triple C patties (see recipe pages 170 and 174), or the Brinner Frittata (see recipe page 184) and that will last us the week. Or if we do get a chance to cook together in the evening, I'll make an easy soup or just stir-fry or bake a bunch of veggies and eat them with a few tablespoons of tahini or hummus.

Dessert After dinner I usually have tea. Some nights I'll have a few squares of dark chocolate or carob, or a tablespoon of almond butter.

Snacks I don't snack a lot, but when I do it might be a green vegetable juice, some veggie sticks or no-salt rice crackers with hummus or a Chief bar (eatlikeachief.com).

THIS WEEK'S (U)NSTOPPABLE FITNESS ACTION
» *Step things up*

It's time to decide on your next move. What will you do next to get even fitter and healthier than you are right now?

We'd love you to join us for the online version of this program at bufgirls.com/totally-buf, which is packed with daily workouts you can do anywhere, right alongside other girls from all corners of the globe. Or if you live close to a BUF Girls outdoor group training location, why not join the movement of Beautiful, Unstoppable, Fearless girls getting fit together in the great Aussie outdoors?

There are so many more options, too - everything from joining a boutique gym to signing up for dance classes, becoming part of a hiking group or training for your first triathlon. Whatever your next move is, make sure you *do* make it. Keep the momentum going and fuel that Unstoppable spirit!

THIS WEEK'S (F)EARLESS MINDSET
» *Develop a growth mindset and never rely on motivation again*

Ever heard of the concept of fixed versus growth mindsets?

Having a fixed mindset means you believe you're either good at something, or not. It means believing you're either smart, or not. When people with a fixed mindset are not good at something, they become frustrated and give up. When they fail, they believe they're no good, and they love it when you tell them they're smart because they believe the abilities they're born with determine everything.

Having a growth mindset means you believe you can learn anything you want to, and that when you feel frustrated you persevere anyway. It means you like to challenge yourself, see failures as learning opportunities and are inspired when you succeed. Someone with a growth mindset likes being told they work hard and believes their effort and attitude determine everything.

A big part of the reason the BUF Girls movement is so special is that our programs are designed around education and empowerment, to help you create a growth mindset. A strict meal plan and a predetermined calorie count won't do that for you, but learning about food, becoming curious about how your body works and focusing on developing a healthy life culture packed with adventure and movement sure will.

If you don't want to rely on motivation to keep you going (and let's be honest, motivation is unreliable), you've got to keep finding ways to stay excited about your healthy path, seeking out new knowledge and experiences that help you to grow.

The first step is to approach it all with the right attitude, and we have a simple trick for this.

REPLACING 'SHOULD' WITH 'WANT'

Whenever you find yourself saying the word 'should', stop and take a moment, then repeat the sentence in your head with the word 'want' in its place.

You can use this for work tasks, social catch-ups, or cooking for the family, but it's incredibly powerful when you use it with the intentions you have for your own health and fitness. For example, 'I should go to the gym today' already feels defeated, but switch one word and it becomes, 'I want to go to the gym today', which automatically makes you feel empowered and like you can't wait to get to the gym. The same goes for 'I should choose a healthier lunch'. How about, 'I want to choose a healthier lunch'?

AFFIRMATIONS FROM OUR FAVOURITE WEIGHT PSYCHOLOGIST

We asked our favourite weight psychologist, Glenn Mackintosh from Weight Management Psychology, to help us out with six beautiful but also practical affirmations based on the journey you've just experienced.

Use these by writing each of them on an individual slip of paper, folding and putting them in a small box. When you're having a moment of self-doubt, bring the box out and reach for a piece of paper. Whatever affirmation you pick up is your back-on-track mantra for the day.

On loving your body: 'Beauty comes in infinite shapes and sizes. Let go of *society's* thin ideal and develop *your own* body standards. **Love your body healthy.**'

On trusting your body: 'Your body is more amazing than you think. It knows when to start eating and when to stop. Listen to your body and you will grow to trust it.'

On listening to your body: 'What foods make you feel energised, light and focused? What foods make you feel tired, slow and foggy? Forget the rules and focus on how food makes you *feel*.'

On creating a healthy body: 'Beautiful, Unstoppable, Fearless girls know they are more than a number on the scales. They are too focused on strength, fitness and function to worry about their weight. Any weight loss is just a bonus of healthy living.'

On respecting your body 'People love to be a part of something positive. Let others in on your intentions, and turn saboteurs into supporters. Respect yourself and others will too.'

On looking after your body long-term: 'Motivation provides the spark, and willpower tends the kindling, but habits fan the flames.'

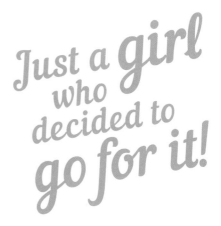

Just a *girl* who decided to *go for it!*

TOP TIPS 'n' TAKEAWAYS

What a ride – you've made it to your very last tips 'n' takeaways list!

Being a BUF Girl is for life. You can't un-learn everything you've soaked up over the past six weeks, so this foodie education will always be with you, and so will our training community of Beautiful, Unstoppable, Fearless women in the online world, or at any of our live training locations around Australia. All you need to do is reach out.

Here's everything you've learned, in one tight list. Take a moment to remember how far you've come since you picked up this book.

» BUF Girls start their days right – eat protein with breakfast, and avoid processed foods and sugar first thing in the morning.

» BUF Girls aren't slaves to sugar – you know how to read labels, are savvy enough to say a confident NO to that office lolly jar, are not afraid of good fats, and try to include protein and veggies at each meal or snack.

» BUF Girls know wholegrains are the best option and that too much of anything is not great, particularly when it comes to inflammatory packaged foods. Mix it up by properly preparing all sorts of scrumptious grains, from nutty brown rice to quinoa, barley, plain oats and buckwheat. You know you can also get a satisfying carbohydrate hit from sweet potato, pumpkin and fruit.

» BUF Girls know the key to a happy tummy is a combo of excellent nutrition, gut-loving and anti-inflammatory foods, plus the right kind of exercise, as well as plenty of rest.

» BUF Girls say a big YES to getting social – you're not scared of the big wide world ruining your health mission. You know that there are healthful choices to be made at most restaurants and events, and if not, understand that a few cheeky treats won't ruin your goals.

» BUF Girls are totally Beautiful, inside and out, Unstoppable thanks to the support of their tribe, and Fearless in going after their goals.

Now that's what we call Totally BUF!

MEAL PLAN

	Breakfast	*Lunch*	*Dinner*
MONDAY	Homemade Bircher Muesli PAGE 113	Apple and Haloumi Salad PAGE 152	Broccoli, Goji and Avocado Salad PAGE 180
TUESDAY	Cheesy Eggs and Greens PAGE 105	Spiced Beef Mince with Kimchi PAGE 172	Sweet Potato Chicken Curry PAGE 220
WEDNESDAY	Sweet Potato Boats with Scrambled Eggs PAGE 122	Egg and Rocket Bruschetta PAGE 133	The 'Orange' Soup PAGE 224
THURSDAY	Breakfast Quinoa PAGE 112	Green Vegetable Loaf PAGE 136	BBQ Chicken and Lime Skewers PAGE 180
FRIDAY	Green Baked Eggs PAGE 114	Quinoa Bake PAGE 153	Vegetable Quinoa Curry PAGE 228

Snack options

» SPINACH BREAD (PAGE 242)
» BAKED EGG MUFFINS (PAGE 235)
» CHOCOLATE MOUSSE (PAGE 234)

Appetite-balance Smoothie

Beautiful
1 handful of spinach leaves
½ cup frozen blueberries

Unstoppable
1 cup milk of your choice, or water
1 serve of protein powder

Fearless
¼ soft avocado
1 tablespoon chia seeds
1 teaspoon maca powder
3 ice cubes

1 Place the milk or water in the blender
   first, then add the remaining ingredients.
   Blend on high until well combined. If you
   prefer a runnier smoothie, simply add a dash
   more water.

Buf Girls' Tip
TOP WITH A HANDFUL OF THE NUTTY
GRANOLA (SEE RECIPE PAGE 116) FOR
AN (U)NSTOPPABLE CARBOHYDRATE
SOURCE BEFORE OR AFTER TRAINING.

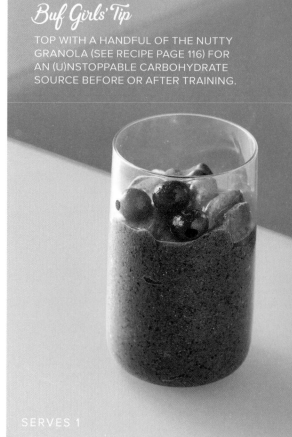

SERVES 1

SERVES 1

Avocado and Feta Smash

Beautiful
1 small red chilli (optional)
1 tablespoon finely chopped coriander leaves
juice of ½ lemon

Unstoppable
1 tablespoon feta (or vegan feta), crumbled
1 slice of bread, toasted, or one serve of
   Oaty Crackers (see recipe page 239)

Fearless
sea salt and pepper, to taste
½ soft avocado
1 tablespoon chia seeds or LSA

1 In a small bowl, mash together the avocado,
   chilli, coriander, lemon juice, feta and salt
   and pepper.
2 Spread the avocado mixture on the toast
   and sprinkle with chia seeds or LSA.

Baked Eggs in Mushrooms

Beautiful
2 portobello mushrooms
1 tablespoon roughly chopped coriander
2 cups roughly chopped spinach leaves

Unstoppable
2 eggs
2 tablespoons feta (or vegan feta), crumbled

Fearless
1 tablespoon olive oil
sea salt and pepper, to taste

1. Preheat the oven to 180°C and line a tray with baking paper.
2. Rinse the mushrooms and remove stalks by carefully cutting away. Place mushrooms on the baking tray and drizzle with the olive oil.
3. Crack an egg into each mushroom and top each with 1 tablespoon feta and a sprinkle of coriander. Season with salt and pepper and place the mushrooms in the oven to cook for 15 minutes.
4. Once cooked, allow to cool slightly, then serve on a bed of spinach.

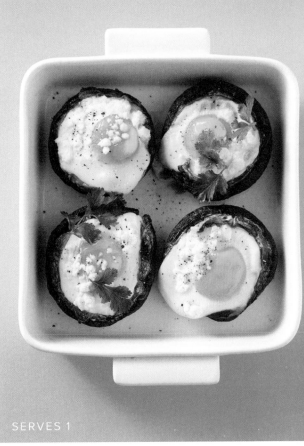

SERVES 1

SERVES 1

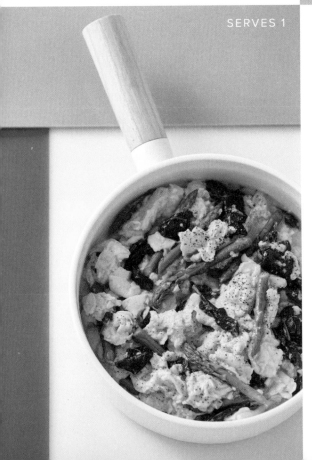

Asparagus Egg Scramble

Beautiful
4 asparagus spears, chopped
1 cup spinach leaves
½ lemon

Unstoppable
2 eggs (or vegan egg substitute)
¼ cup almond milk

Fearless
1 tablespoon coconut oil
sea salt and pepper, to taste

1. Crack the eggs into a bowl, add the almond milk and season with salt and pepper. Whisk until light and fluffy.
2. Place a frying pan over medium heat, add the coconut oil and pour the egg mixture into the pan. Once the eggs begin to cook, add the asparagus and spinach and begin to scramble the egg mixture. Cook to your liking, then remove from the pan, squeeze over the lemon juice and season with extra salt and pepper, if desired.

Basic Omelette

Beautiful

1 cup roughly chopped spinach
   leaves
1 cup green veggies of your choice
   (e.g. broccoli, kale, green beans,
   peas)
1 teaspoon chilli flakes
½ lemon (optional)

Unstoppable

2 eggs (or vegan egg substitute)
1 slice of sourdough bread,
   toasted (optional)

Fearless

1 tablespoon chia seeds
1 tablespoon coconut oil
sea salt and pepper, to taste

1   Crack the eggs into a bowl, add the chia seeds
    and salt and pepper and whisk until well
    combined.

2   Heat the oil in a frying pan over medium heat
    and pour in the egg mixture. Allow to cook for
    2 minutes, or until the egg starts to bubble, then
    top with spinach and vegetables of your choice.

3   Season well and cover with a lid for quicker
    cooking. Allow to cook for another 3 minutes,
    or until the egg is cooked to your liking.

4   Carefully remove the omelette from the pan,
    sprinkle with chilli flakes, squeeze the lemon
    over, if using, and serve on its own, or with
    sourdough toast or a slice of Spinach Bread
    (see recipe page 242).

SERVES 1

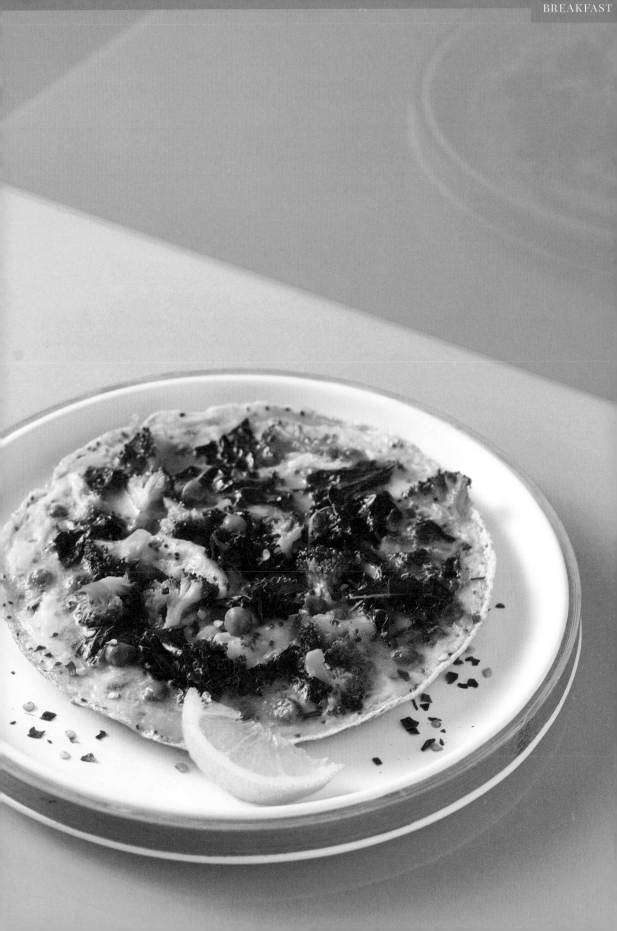

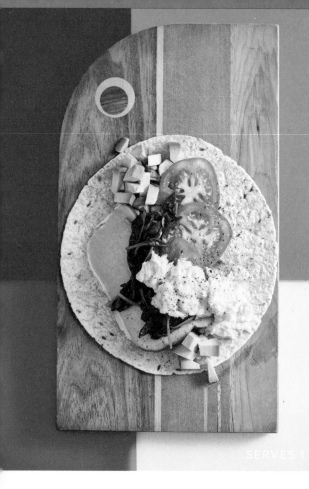

Breakfast Tortilla

Beautiful
2 cups spinach leaves
1 tomato, sliced

Unstoppable
1 egg (or vegan egg substitute)
1 small tortilla wrap
50 g ham off the bone (optional)

Fearless
1 tablespoon coconut oil
¼–½ avocado
sea salt and pepper, to taste

1 To cook the egg, heat the coconut oil in a frying pan and crack the egg into the pan. Cook to your liking then remove from the pan.

2 Add the spinach to the same pan with a dash of water, and cook until wilted.

3 Spread the avocado on the wrap then top with tomato, wilted spinach, fried egg and ham, if using. Season with salt and pepper.

SERVES 1

Bubble and Squeak

Beautiful
2 cups spinach leaves
½ cup Cinnamon Roasted Pumpkin
   (see recipe page 242)
½ lemon

Unstoppable
1 egg (or vegan egg substitute)
1 rasher of bacon or ham (optional)
50 g (2 slices) haloumi (or vegan feta)

Fearless
1 tablespoon coconut oil
¼–½ avocado
sea salt and pepper, to taste

1 Heat the coconut oil in a frying pan and fry the bacon and haloumi until lightly browned. Flip the haloumi halfway through. While the bacon and haloumi are cooking, make room in the pan and crack in the egg.

2 Once the egg, bacon and haloumi are cooked, remove from the pan. Serve on a bed of spinach with Cinnamon Roasted Pumpkin and the avocado. Season with salt and pepper and a squeeze of lemon juice.

SERVES 1

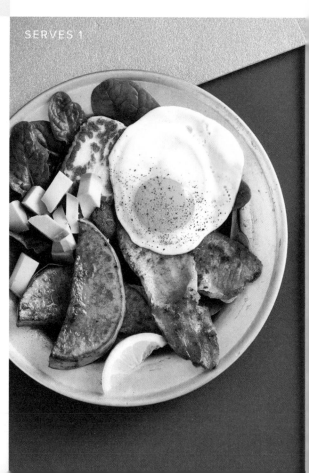

Vegan option

REPLACE THE EGG WITH TEMPEH
OR A VEGAN EGG SUBSTITUTE.

Cheesy Eggs and Greens

Beautiful
1 spring onion, sliced
1 zucchini, chopped
1 cup dark leafy greens (e.g. silverbeet, chard,
    spinach, kale), stalks removed and leaves chopped

Unstoppable
4 eggs

Fearless
2 tablespoons coconut oil
splash of apple cider vinegar
2 teaspoons nutritional yeast flakes
sea salt and pepper, to taste

1 Melt the oil in a saucepan over medium-high heat.
  Add the spring onion and stir until soft. Add the
  zucchini and cook until just soft.

2 Turn the heat to low-medium and add the remaining
  greens and a little apple cider vinegar. Cook until the
  greens are wilted.

3 Turn the heat to low and add the eggs, stirring
  frequently to avoid them sticking to the pan. When the
  eggs are just cooked, add the nutritional yeast flakes
  and salt and pepper to taste, and stir to combine.

SERVES 2

SERVES 1

Carrot Cake Oats

Beautiful
1 carrot, grated

Unstoppable
⅓ cup rolled oats
1 tablespoon protein powder of your choice
1 Medjool date, chopped
1 tablespoon chopped walnuts

Fearless
1 cup coconut milk
1½ teaspoons cinnamon
¼ teaspoon nutmeg

1 Place the carrot, oats, coconut milk, protein,
  1 teaspoon of the cinnamon and the nutmeg in a
  saucepan. Cook over medium heat for 2–3 minutes,
  or until the oats have absorbed the liquid.

2 Top with the date and walnuts and sprinkle with
  the remaining cinnamon.

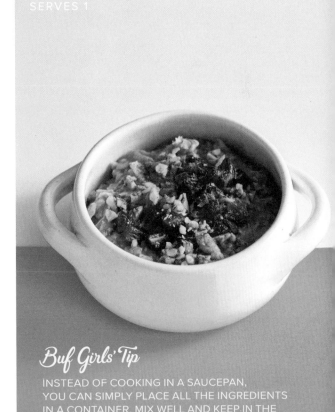

Buf Girls' Tip

INSTEAD OF COOKING IN A SAUCEPAN,
YOU CAN SIMPLY PLACE ALL THE INGREDIENTS
IN A CONTAINER, MIX WELL AND KEEP IN THE
FRIDGE OVERNIGHT.

Chia Pudding with Almonds and Goji Berries

Beautiful

½ cup frozen or fresh blueberries,
　　to serve

1 tablespoon goji berries, to serve

Unstoppable

¾ cup milk of your choice
　　(e.g. almond or coconut)

1 tablespoon almonds
　　(about 12 almonds)

1 serve of protein powder

Fearless

¼ cup chia seeds

½ teaspoon cinnamon

½ teaspoon vanilla essence

1　Place milk, chia seeds, almonds, cinnamon, vanilla and protein powder in a blender and whiz for 15 seconds, or until combined (the texture should resemble a pudding). TIP: add the liquid before you put the chia seeds in, to avoid them sticking to the bottom of the blender!

2　Pour the mixture into a small container or jar (or keep in the blender) and place in the fridge overnight to set.

3　When ready to eat, top with blueberries and goji berries.

SERVES 1

Buf Girls' Tip

YOU CAN SUBSTITUTE
THE BLUEBERRIES FOR
THE SAME QUANTITY
OF RASPBERRIES OR
HALF A BANANA.

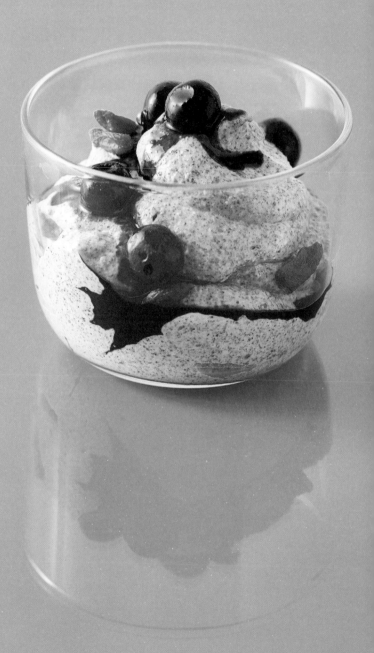

Coco Quinoa Bowl

Beautiful
1 tablespoon raisins or chopped dried figs
1 cup fresh blueberries, to serve

Unstoppable
¾ cup quinoa
2 tablespoons walnuts (or nuts of your choice)
1–2 teaspoons stevia or honey

Fearless
500 ml water
½–1 cup coconut milk
2 tablespoons coconut yoghurt, to serve
¼ teaspoon cinnamon

1 Rinse the quinoa really well, add the water and bring to the boil. Add a little more water if needed. Reduce the heat to medium-low and cook, covered, for 10 minutes.

2 Stir in half the coconut milk and the dried fruit and nuts. Cook, covered, for another 10 minutes, then stir in the stevia or honey, the cinnamon and the remaining milk.

3 Serve with blueberries and a dollop of yoghurt on top.

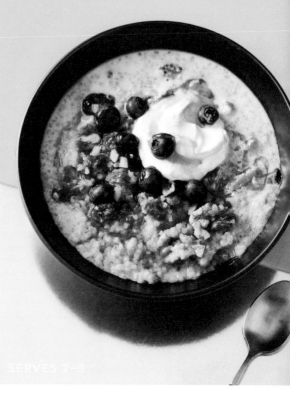

SERVES 2–3

SERVES 1

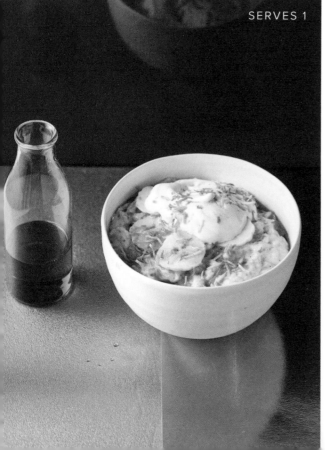

Coconut Porridge

Beautiful
½ banana, sliced

Unstoppable
⅓ cup rolled oats
1 cup coconut milk
1 tablespoon maple syrup
2 tablespoons natural yoghurt or coconut yoghurt

Fearless
¼ cup shredded coconut
1 teaspoon cinnamon
½ tablespoon psyllium husks

1 Heat a saucepan over medium heat and toast the shredded coconut until golden. Add the oats, coconut milk, cinnamon and psyllium husks. Cook for 2–3 minutes, or until the oats have absorbed the liquid.

2 Top with sliced banana, a drizzle of maple syrup and yoghurt of your choice.

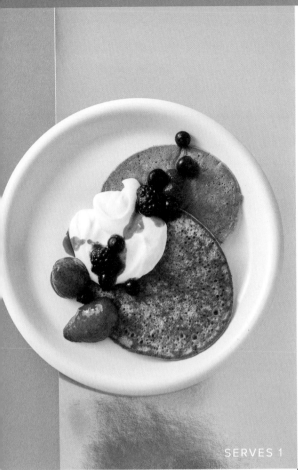

Easy Peasy Protein Pancakes

Beautiful
1 banana
½ cup frozen berries, thawed, to serve

Unstoppable
2 eggs (or vegan egg substitute)

Fearless
1 tablespoon butter or coconut oil
1 teaspoon cinnamon
pinch of nutmeg
coconut yoghurt, or toppings of your choice

1. Place the banana, eggs, cinnamon and nutmeg in a blender and whiz until combined.
2. Pour into a lightly oiled or buttered pan and cook as you would regular pancakes. Recipe makes one large, or two small, pancakes.
3. Serve with your topping/s of choice.

SERVES 1

Failsafe Breakfast Salad

Beautiful
1 Roma tomato
2 sprigs of rosemary
1 handful of spinach leaves
mint leaves, to taste
   (we like about 6, chopped)
¼ red onion, diced, or a handful of sliced
   spring onion

Unstoppable
2 eggs, poached

Fearless
sea salt and pepper, to taste
diced black olives, to serve (optional)

1. Cut the tomato in half, sprinkle with rosemary and salt and cook under a low grill until soft.
2. Place the tomatoes on a plate with the spinach, mint and onion, top with poached eggs and, if you like, diced black olives. Serve and enjoy.

SERVES 1

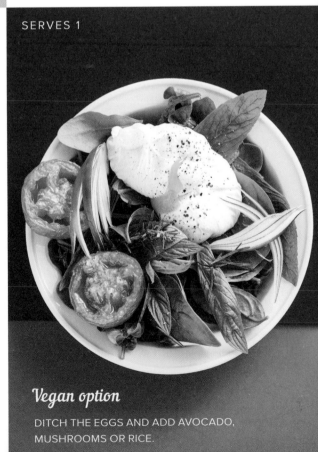

Vegan option
DITCH THE EGGS AND ADD AVOCADO, MUSHROOMS OR RICE.

Fried Eggs with Almond Butter Greens

Beautiful

1 cup chopped broccoli
½ zucchini, thinly sliced
½ cup peas, fresh or frozen
1 teaspoon chilli flakes
juice of ½ lemon

Unstoppable

2 eggs
1 cup of roasted veggies
   (e.g. Cinnamon Roasted Pumpkin
   – see recipe page 242)
1 tablespoon almond butter

Fearless

1 tablespoon coconut oil
sea salt and pepper, to taste

1 To cook the eggs, heat half of the coconut oil in a frying pan over medium heat and crack eggs into the pan. Top eggs with the chilli flakes and cook to your liking. Remove from the pan.

2 To cook your vegetables, heat the remaining coconut oil in the pan and add the broccoli, zucchini and peas. Sauté until softened (add a dash of water to help sauté the veggies).

3 Remove the greens from the pan and drizzle with the almond butter and top with eggs. Season with lemon juice, salt and pepper. Serve with a side of Cinnamon Roasted Pumpkin (see recipe page 242).

SERVES 1

Vegan option

DITCH THE EGGS AND JUST EAT MORE VEGGIES, PERHAPS EVEN SPRINKLED WITH NUTS, OR DRIZZLED WITH TAHINI.

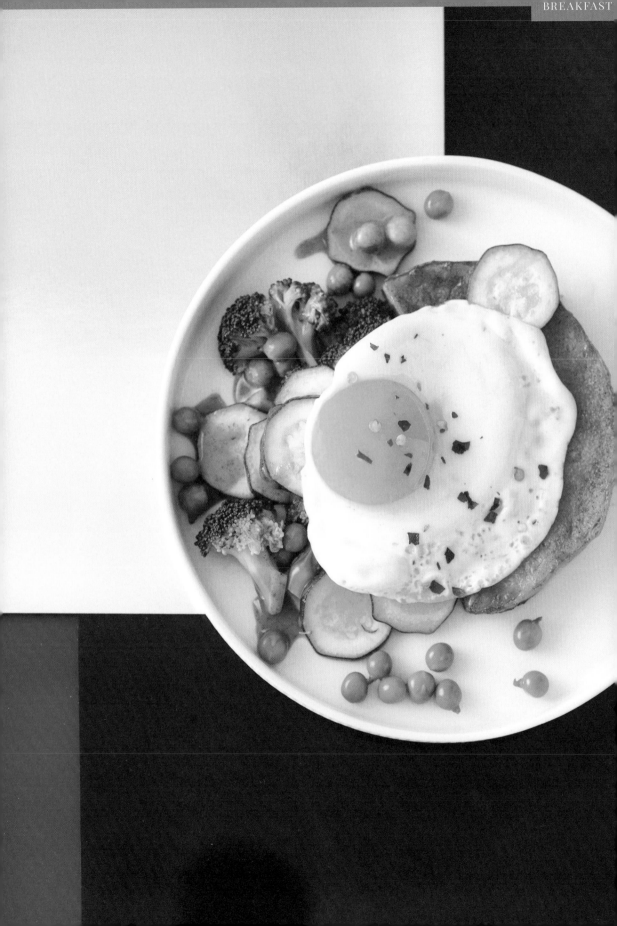

Glow Juice

2 kale leaves
handful of spinach leaves
¼ lemon
½ apple
1 cucumber
1 celery stick
1 handful of chia seeds

1 Feed the ingredients through your juicer, or just chop and whiz them up in a blender and enjoy!

Buf Girls' Tip

WHEN IT COMES TO A GOOD GREEN JUICE, THERE ARE ESSENTIALLY THREE FLAVOURS OF LEAFY GREENS: NEUTRAL ONES LIKE LETTUCE; EARTHY ONES LIKE CHARD AND KALE; AND PEPPERY ONES LIKE MUSTARD AND DANDELION. NEUTRAL ARE EASIER TO WORK WITH, SO START WITH THEM.

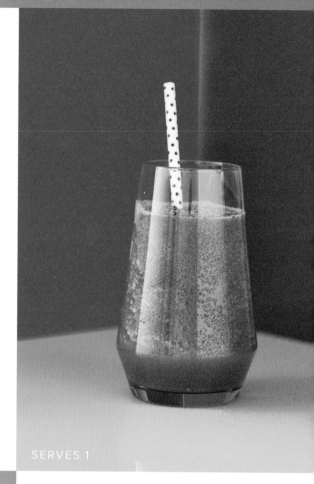

SERVES 1

SERVES 1

Buf Girls' Tip

TOP WITH A HANDFUL OF THE NUTTY GRANOLA (SEE RECIPE PAGE 116) FOR AN (U)NSTOPPABLE CARBOHYDRATE SOURCE BEFORE OR AFTER TRAINING.

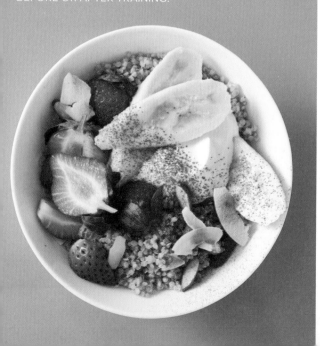

Breakfast Quinoa

Beautiful
½ banana, sliced
½ cup hulled, sliced strawberries

Unstoppable
½ cup cooked quinoa
¼ cup roughly chopped almonds
(or seeds of your choice)
natural or coconut yoghurt, to serve (optional)

Fearless
1 tablespoon coconut flakes
1 teaspoon cinnamon

1 Combine all the ingredients in a bowl, mix well and enjoy!

Green Smoothie Bowl

Beautiful
½ Lebanese cucumber, cut into small chunks
½ cup frozen mixed berries
½ frozen banana
1 handful of kale (or other greens), roughly chopped
1 kiwifruit, sliced, to serve

Unstoppable
1 cup milk of your choice
1 serve of protein powder
1 tablespoon LSA, to serve

Fearless
½ tablespoon psyllium husks
3 ice cubes
1 tablespoon chia seeds, to serve

1 Pour the milk into the blender, then add the cucumber, berries, banana, kale, protein powder, psyllium husks and ice cubes. Whiz on high until well combined.
2 Pour the smoothie into a bowl and top with kiwifruit, LSA and chia seeds.

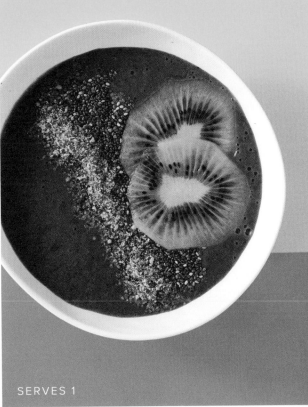

SERVES 1

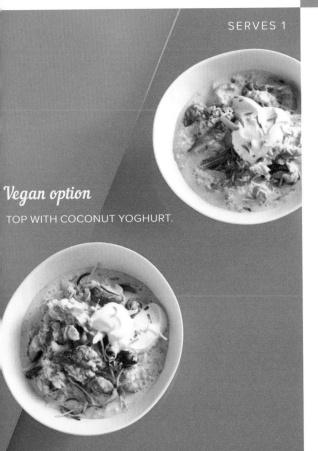

SERVES 1

Vegan option
TOP WITH COCONUT YOGHURT.

Homemade Bircher Muesli

Beautiful
½ green apple

Unstoppable
⅓ cup rolled oats
1 small handful of activated mixed nuts
250 ml milk of your choice, plus extra for serving
¼ cup yoghurt of your choice, to serve

Fearless
pinch of salt
1 teaspoon honey or maple syrup
1 teaspoon cinnamon, to serve
1 small handful of shredded coconut, to serve

1 The night before you want to eat the bircher muesli, soak the oats and nuts with the milk and salt. Stir well and put the bowl in the fridge.
2 In the morning, grab the oats, stir in the honey, if using, and grate the apple on top. Dollop on the yoghurt and sprinkle with cinnamon and coconut.

Green Baked Eggs

Beautiful

½ leek, sliced

1 clove garlic, crushed

1 zucchini, sliced

½ cup sliced mushrooms

3 kale leaves, stalks removed and leaves chopped

Unstoppable

2 eggs

Fearless

1 tablespoon coconut oil

½ teaspoon ground coriander

½ teaspoon ground cumin

chilli flakes (optional)

sea salt and pepper, to taste

crumbled goat's or sheep's feta, to serve (optional)

sliced avocado, to serve

1   Preheat the oven to 160°C.

2   Place an ovenproof frying pan over medium heat, add the coconut oil and sauté the leek and garlic until golden brown. Add the spices and salt, toss in the zucchini, mushrooms and kale and cook for 6–7 minutes, or until the vegetables have softened.

3   Push everything to the side of the pan to make room for the eggs. Crack the eggs in.

4   Pop the pan into the oven and allow to cook for 10 minutes, or until the eggs have set.

5   Remove the pan from the oven, sprinkle with crumbled feta, avocado and pepper, and serve.

SERVES 1

Vegan option

ADD 2–3 BIG SPOONFULS OF HUMMUS IN PLACE OF THE EGGS BEFORE BAKING.

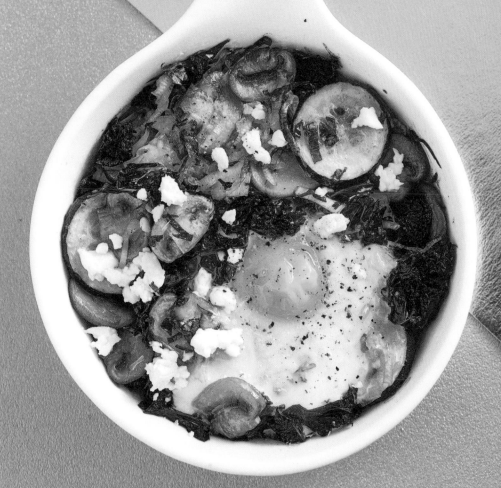

'Buf Girls' fave!

Nutty Granola

Beautiful

1 cup activated buckwheat groats
½ cup roughly chopped dried dates

Unstoppable

1 cup rolled oats
½ cup roughly chopped almonds
½ cup pecans
¼ cup peanut butter
¼ cup rice malt syrup

Fearless

½ cup coconut flakes
1 teaspoon cinnamon
½ teaspoon sea salt
2 tablespoons coconut oil
1 teaspoon vanilla essence

1   Preheat the oven to 160°C and line a large tray with baking paper.

2   Place the oats, buckwheat groats, almonds, pecans, dates, coconut flakes, cinnamon and salt in a bowl and mix to combine.

3   Place the peanut butter, rice malt syrup, coconut oil and vanilla in a small saucepan and cook over low heat for 2–3 minutes, or until the mixture is combined.

4   Pour the wet mixture into the dry ingredients and mix until evenly coated.

5   Pour granola onto the tray and bake for 15 minutes. Remove the tray at the 10-minute mark and stir the mixture to ensure it's evenly cooked before returning to the oven to cook for a final 5 minutes.

6   Allow to cool completely on the tray, then store in an airtight container.

SERVES 6

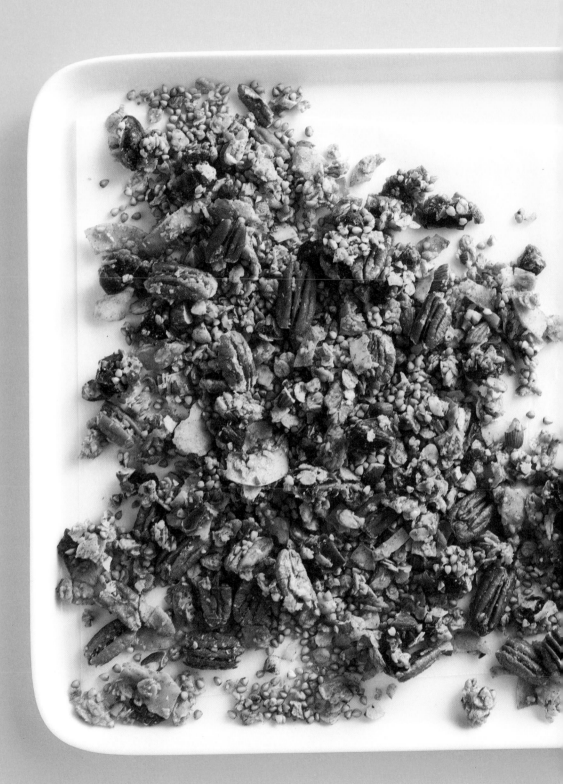

Pumpkin, Spinach and Feta Breakfast Muffins

Beautiful

1½ cups grated pumpkin

1 cup roughly chopped spinach
  leaves

½ cup roughly chopped parsley

Unstoppable

¾ cup almond meal

1 cup buckwheat flour

3 eggs (or vegan substitute)

½ cup almond milk

100 g feta (or vegan feta),
  crumbled

¼ cup almonds, roughly chopped

Fearless

1 teaspoon cinnamon

1 tablespoon chia seeds

1 teaspoon baking powder

1 teaspoon sea salt

¼ cup coconut oil

1 Preheat the oven to 180°C and line a muffin tin with patty cases.

2 In a large bowl, mix together the almond meal, buckwheat flour, cinnamon, chia seeds, baking powder and salt.

3 In a separate bowl, mix together the eggs, almond milk and coconut oil.

4 Add the dry mixture to the wet mixture, then add the pumpkin, spinach, parsley and feta.

5 Scoop the batter into the patty cases, top with almonds and bake for 25 minutes, or until cooked through.

SERVES 8

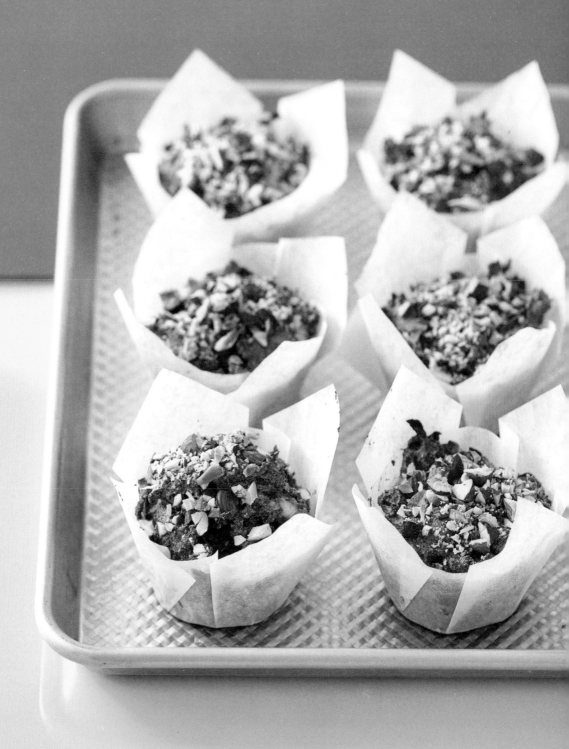

Veggie Quinoa Bowl

Beautiful

1 cup chopped broccoli
2 cups roughly chopped kale
1 cup spinach leaves
½ Lebanese cucumber, diced
½ lemon

Unstoppable

½ cup quinoa (yields 1½ cups
   of cooked quinoa)
1–2 boiled eggs
2 tablespoons Avocado and
   Chickpea Hummus
   (see recipe page 243)

Fearless

1 tablespoon coconut oil
¼–½ avocado, sliced
1 tablespoon apple cider vinegar
sea salt and pepper, to taste

1 Heat the oil in a frying pan and add the broccoli
and kale. Sauté for 3-4 minutes, or until the kale
is wilted.

2 To cook the quinoa, place it in a saucepan, add
1 cup of water and bring to the boil. Once boiling,
turn the heat down to a simmer and cook with
the lid on for 15 minutes, or until the water has
absorbed and quinoa is cooked.

3 To construct your bowl, arrange the cooked
broccoli and kale, spinach, cucumber, boiled
eggs, quinoa and avocado in a bowl. Season
with salt and pepper and finish with a drizzle
of apple cider vinegar, Avocado Hummus and
a squeeze of lemon juice.

SERVES 1

Vegan option

REPLACE THE EGGS
WITH A STORE-BOUGHT
FELAFEL OR TWO.

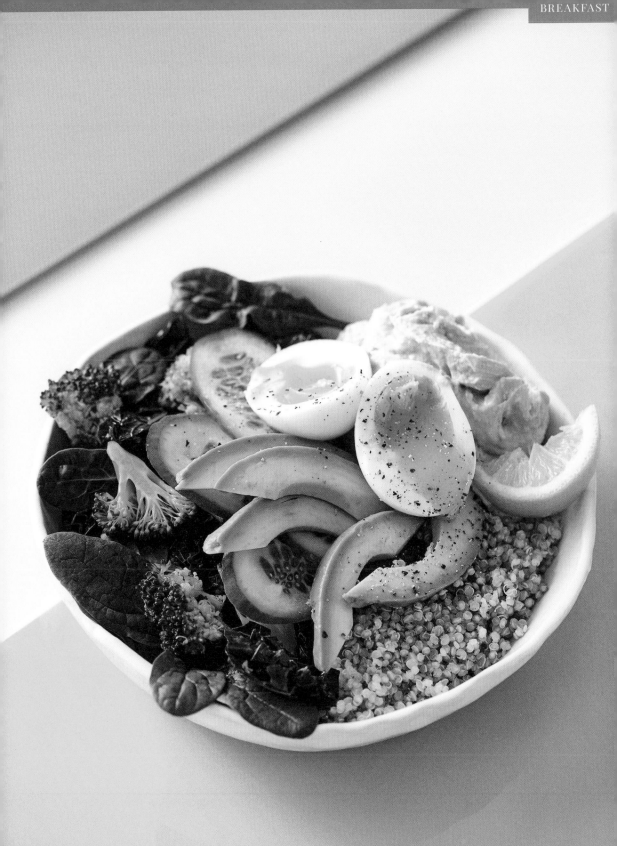

Sweet Potato Boats with Scrambled Eggs

Beautiful

1 small sweet potato, cut in half
2 cups spinach leaves
1 tablespoon roughly chopped
   coriander
½ lemon

Unstoppable

2 eggs, beaten

Fearless

2 tablespoons olive oil
sea salt and pepper, to taste
½ avocado

1   Preheat the oven to 180°C and line a tray with baking paper.

2   Rub 1 tablespoon of the oil onto the sweet potato halves and sprinkle with salt. Place cut-sides down on the tray and bake for 20 minutes, or until softened.

3   Once the sweet potato is almost cooked, heat a frying pan with the remaining oil and pour the beaten egg into the pan. Once the egg begins to cook, add the spinach and scramble the mixture. Cook to your liking then remove from the pan.

4   Place one sweet potato half onto a plate and top with the avocado, scrambled eggs and a sprinkle of coriander. Squeeze over some lemon juice and season with salt and pepper.

SERVES 1

Vegan option

SUBSTITUTE THE EGG FOR
SCRAMBLED SILKEN TOFU,
OR MIXED BEANS.

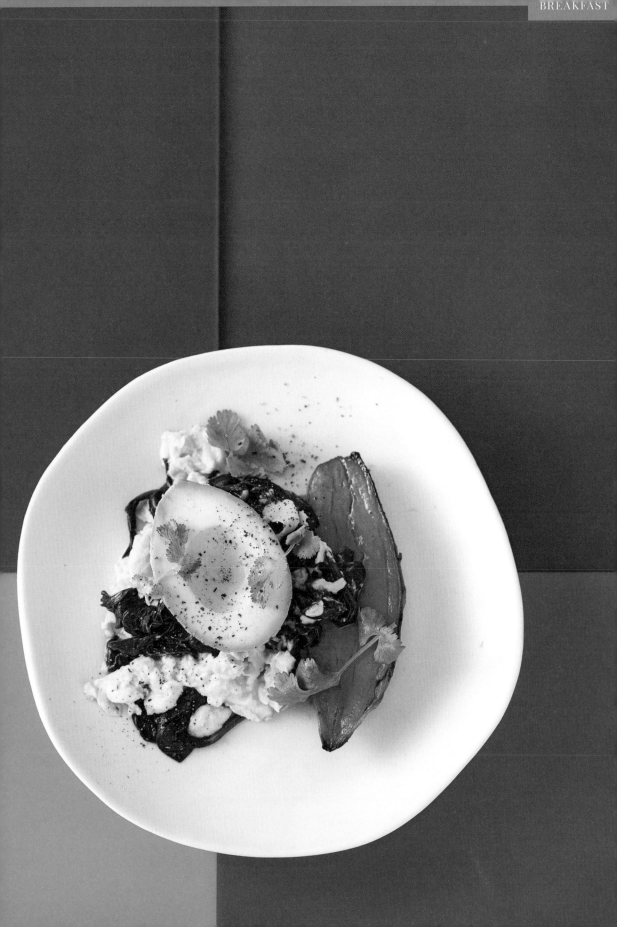

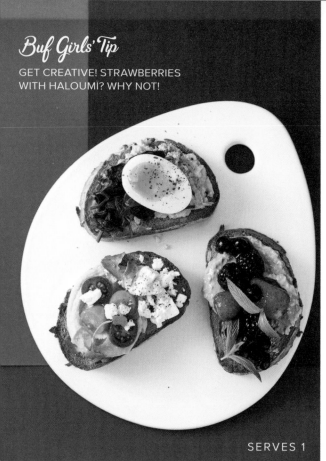

Toast Toppers

Beautiful

vegetables of your choice (e.g. cucumber,
   sliced tomato, wilted or fresh spinach)
fruits of your choice (e.g. banana, berries)

Unstoppable

1–2 eggs
50 g haloumi
2 tablespoons hummus
2 tablespoons crumbled feta
nuts and seeds of your choice
1–2 slices of bread

Fearless

½ avocado
1–2 tablespoons nut butter

1 Top your choice of bread with any
  (B) veg/fruit, (U) protein/carb + (F) fat, such as:

- spinach + egg + avocado

- tomato + haloumi + avocado

- berries + almond butter

Naked Breakfast Bowl

Beautiful

2 handfuls of spinach leaves
6 cherry tomatoes, halved
½ lemon

Unstoppable

2 eggs
1 tablespoon crumbled feta
1 tablespoon roughly chopped
   dry-roasted almonds

Fearless

¼ avocado, sliced
sea salt and pepper, to taste

1 Carefully place eggs in a saucepan of boiling water and
  allow to boil for 3 minutes. Cool, peel and cut in half.

2 To prepare your breakfast bowl, fill the bottom
  of the bowl with spinach leaves, then top with the
  cherry tomatoes, avocado, feta and almonds, and
  place your halved eggs on top.

3 Season with a squeeze of lemon juice and salt and
  pepper.

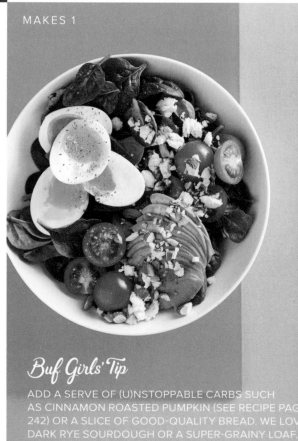

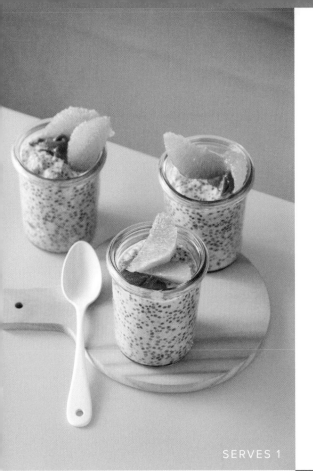

SERVES 1

Vanilla Orange Overnight Proats

Beautiful
1 tablespoon orange zest
½ orange, peeled and cut into small chunks

Unstoppable
⅓ cup rolled oats
¾ cup almond milk
1 serve of protein powder
1 tablespoon nut butter (e.g. almond or cashew)

Fearless
1 tablespoon chia seeds
1 teaspoon vanilla essence

1 The day or night before, in a bowl or jar, combine the oats, almond milk, protein powder, orange zest, chia seeds and vanilla. Allow the mixture to stand on the bench for 10 minutes, then stir once before placing in the fridge.

2 The next morning, give the oats a stir and top with orange (or other low-sugar fruit of your choice – e.g. berries or citrus) and a dollop of nut butter.

Very Vegetable Fritters

Beautiful
1 cup grated zucchini
1 cup peas, fresh or frozen
1 handful of roughly chopped parsley
  (or swap for kale)
1 handful of roughly chopped mint
2 spring onions, sliced

Unstoppable
2–3 eggs (or vegan substitute)
½ cup almond meal

Fearless
sea salt and pepper, to taste
1 tablespoon coconut oil

Grate the zucchini then squeeze out as much moisture as you can. Place in a bowl and add the peas, parsley, mint, spring onions, salt, pepper, eggs and almond meal. Mix well and shape into patties.

Place a frying pan over medium heat, add the coconut oil and cook the fritters for 2 minutes each side, or until golden brown.

SERVES 1–2

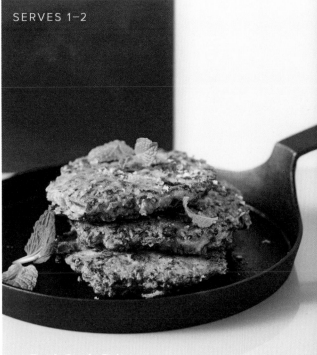

Buf Girls' Tip
THESE ARE GREAT TO MAKE IN BIG BATCHES AND FREEZE FOR WHEN YOU HAVEN'T PLANNED A MEAL.

Quinoa Cacao Muesli

Beautiful

½ cup pepitas

Unstoppable

1½ cups rolled oats

1 cup puffed quinoa

½ cup roughly chopped cashews

¼ cup maple syrup

½ cup goji berries

Fearless

½ cup desiccated coconut

¼ cup cacao powder

1 teaspoon sea salt

¼ cup coconut oil

½ cup tahini

1   Preheat the oven to 180°C and line a large tray with baking paper.

2   Place the oats, quinoa, cashews, pepitas, desiccated coconut, cacao and salt in a bowl and mix to combine.

3   Place the maple syrup, coconut oil and tahini in a small saucepan and cook over low heat for 2–3 minutes, or until the mixture is combined.

4   Pour the wet mixture into the dry ingredients and mix until evenly coated.

5   Pour granola onto the tray and bake for 15 minutes. Remove the tray at the 10-minute mark and stir the mixture to ensure it's evenly cooked. Return to the oven to cook for a final 5 minutes.

6   Allow to cool completely on the tray, then stir in the goji berries and store in an airtight container.

SERVES 1

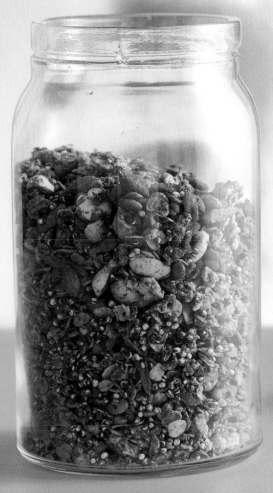
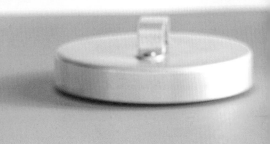

Sautéed Greens Bowl

Beautiful

½ bunch broccolini, finely chopped

1 kale leaf, stalk removed and leaf
   roughly chopped

4 button mushrooms, quartered

2 handfuls of spinach leaves

½ lemon

Unstoppable

2 eggs

1 slice sourdough (optional)

Fearless

1 teaspoon apple cider vinegar
   (for poaching)

¼ avocado, sliced

1 tablespoon coconut oil

sea salt and pepper, to taste

1 To poach eggs, fill a saucepan with water, bring to the boil and add the vinegar. Crack one egg at a time into a cup. Before tipping each egg into the water, create a slow whirlpool with a spoon. Carefully tip in the egg and cook for approximately 3 minutes, or until cooked to your liking. Once the eggs are cooked, remove with a slotted spoon and drain excess water onto a paper towel. Option: you can boil your eggs, if you prefer!

2 To cook the vegetables, place a large frying pan over medium heat and add the coconut oil. Add the broccolini, kale and mushrooms and sauté until softened, then add the spinach and stir until just wilted. Transfer the greens to your serving bowl.

3 Carefully place the poached eggs on the greens and add the sliced avocado on top.

4 To finish, season with freshly squeezed lemon juice, salt and pepper. Serve with a side of sourdough, if you like.

SERVES 1

Vegan option

REPLACE THE EGGS
WITH A TABLESPOON OF
TAHINI AND A SPRINKLE
OF PINE NUTS.

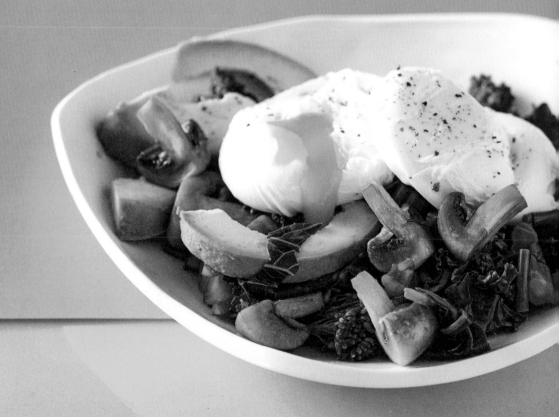

Bacon and Broccoli Salad

Beautiful

2 heads of broccoli

½ red onion, thinly sliced

Unstoppable

4 rashers of bacon, diced

½ cup flaked almonds

Fearless

YOGHURT DRESSING

juice of ½ lemon

½ cup natural yoghurt

2 tablespoons tahini

1 tablespoon apple cider vinegar

1 teaspoon sea salt

1 teaspoon maple syrup

1 Finely dice the broccoli and place in a bowl with the red onion and flaked almonds.

2 Place a frying pan over medium heat and add the bacon. Cook, stirring often, for 5 minutes, or until the bacon is golden brown.

3 Remove the bacon from the pan, allow to cool slightly, then add to the bowl with the broccoli and onion.

4 To make the Yoghurt Dressing, place all the dressing ingredients in a small bowl and mix until well combined.

5 Pour the dressing over the broccoli and bacon mixture and fold through until the salad is evenly coated.

SERVES 4

Vegan option

SUBSTITUTE COCONUT YOGHURT FOR THE NATURAL YOGHURT. ALSO TRY REPLACING THE BACON WITH THINLY SLICED PAN-FRIED TEMPEH, OR PAN-TOSSED SEEDS/NUTS AND CROUTONS (JUST CUBE SOME GRAINY BREAD AND FRY IN THE PAN!).

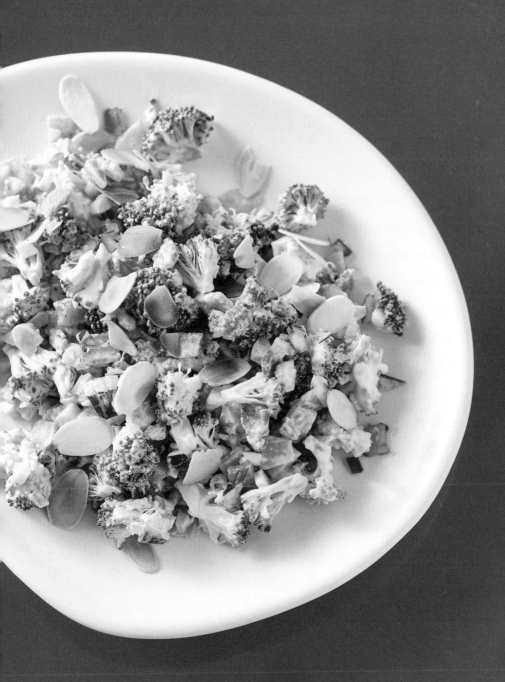

Avocado and Strawberry Salad

Beautiful
1 punnet of strawberries, trimmed and cut into
  quarters
2 cups rocket
juice of ½ lemon

Unstoppable
¼ cup pepitas

Fearless
1 avocado, sliced
1 tablespoon olive oil
2 tablespoons balsamic vinegar
sea salt and pepper, to taste

1 Heat a frying pan over medium heat and dry-fry
   the pepitas. Remove when they start to pop.
2 Toss the strawberries, rocket and avocado
   together in a bowl. Dress with the lemon juice, olive
   oil, balsamic vinegar and a little salt and pepper,
   and mix.
3 Sprinkle the salad with the toasted pepitas and
   it's ready to serve.

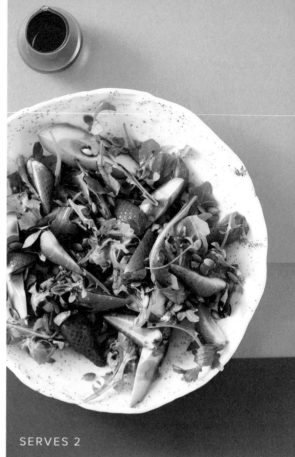

SERVES 2

SERVES 2

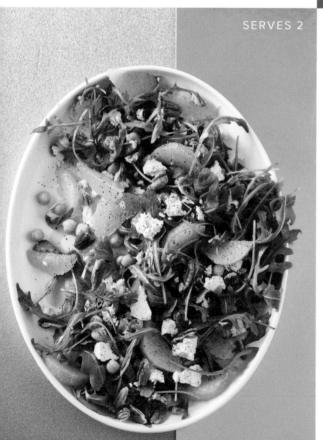

Chickpea, Orange and Goat's Feta Salad

Beautiful
1 orange, peeled and cut into
  small chunks
2 cups rocket

Unstoppable
200 g (½ can) cooked chickpeas, drained
  and rinsed
70 g goat's feta (or vegan feta)
2 tablespoons roughly chopped pecans

Fearless
½ tablespoon olive oil
sea salt and pepper, to taste

1 In a large bowl, combine the orange, rocket,
   chickpeas, feta and pecans. Toss to combine,
   then dress with olive oil and season with
   salt and pepper.

Cucumber 'Fresh As' Salad

Beautiful
2 Lebanese cucumbers, thinly sliced
2 cups rocket
½ cup peas, fresh or frozen
¼ cup roughly chopped dill
juice of ½ lemon

Unstoppable
2 tablespoons crumbled goat's feta

Fearless
1 tablespoon olive oil
1 tablespoon apple cider vinegar
sea salt and pepper, to taste

Toss the cucumber, rocket, peas and dill together in a bowl.

To make the dressing, simply combine the lemon juice, olive oil and vinegar and whisk together.

Top the salad with goat's feta, pour the dressing over and season with salt and pepper.

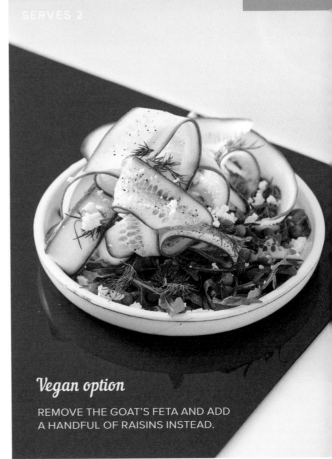

Vegan option
REMOVE THE GOAT'S FETA AND ADD A HANDFUL OF RAISINS INSTEAD.

Egg and Rocket Bruschetta

Beautiful
1 tomato, sliced
1 handful of rocket

Unstoppable
2 boiled eggs (or 2 tablespoons hummus)
1 slice of bread

Fearless
¼–½ avocado, mashed
sea salt and pepper, to taste
1 teaspoon chilli flakes (optional)

1 In a bowl, mash together the boiled eggs and avocado and season with a little salt and pepper.

2 Spread the egg and avocado mixture onto the bread and top with the tomato, rocket and, if you like, chilli flakes.

Grated Salad with Tahini Dressing

Beautiful

1 carrot
1 zucchini
1 beetroot

Unstoppable

½ cup nuts and seeds of your
  choice (e.g. flaked almonds
  and sunflower seeds)

Fearless

TAHINI DRESSING

  juice of ½ lemon
  2 tablespoons tahini
  1 tablespoon olive oil
  1 tablespoon water
  1 teaspoon apple cider vinegar
  ½ teaspoon sea salt

1 Wash the vegetables well, then grate and
   combine in a large bowl.

2 Heat a small frying pan over medium heat and
   dry-fry the nuts and seeds. Remove from the
   pan when lightly golden.

3 To make the Tahini Dressing, simply combine all
   dressing ingredients in a small jug and mix well.

4 Pour the dressing onto the grated vegetables
   and toss to combine. Mix through the nuts and
   the salad is ready to go.

SERVES 2

Buf Girls' Tip

YOU COULD PAIR THIS
WITH AN EXTRA SERVE OF
PROTEIN (CHICKEN, EGGS,
TEMPEH) AND/OR A SERVE
OF LEFTOVER QUINOA
OR BROWN RICE TOSSED
THROUGH.

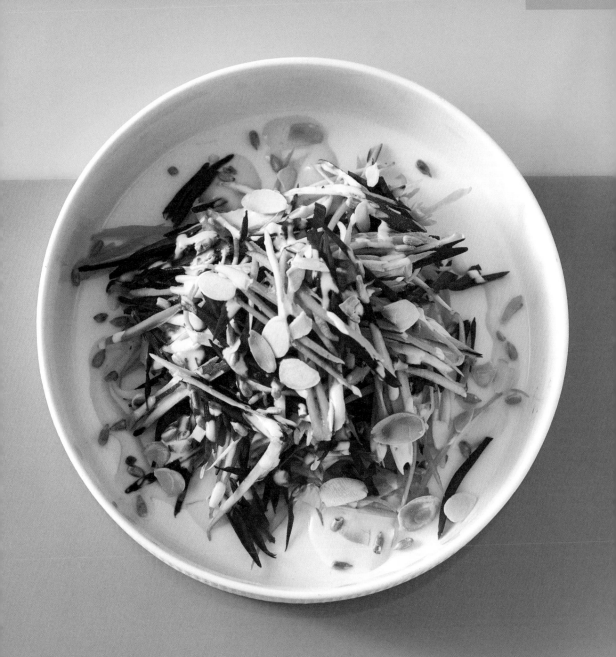

Green Vegetable Loaf

Beautiful

2 cups grated zucchini

2 cups grated carrot

2 cups finely chopped spinach leaves

2 cups finely chopped kale leaves

2 tablespoons chopped basil

2 tablespoons chopped parsley

Unstoppable

3 tablespoons flax seeds

6 eggs

⅔ cup chickpea flour

2 tablespoons sesame seeds

3 tablespoons grated Parmesan or nutritional yeast flakes

⅓ cup pepitas

Fearless

1 tablespoon coconut oil

½ teaspoon ground coriander

½ teaspoon ground cumin

pinch of chilli flakes (optional)

½ teaspoon sea salt

pepper, to taste

1 Mix the flax seeds with ⅓ cup of water and leave to 'gel' for 15 minutes. Place the grated zucchini and carrot on paper towels to drain off excess water.

2 Preheat the oven to 180°C and line the base and sides of a loaf tin with baking paper. Allow the paper to extend over the sides.

3 Combine the spinach, kale, basil and parsley in a large bowl.

4 Whisk together the eggs and season with salt and pepper. Stir the eggs through the green mix. Next, add the carrot, zucchini, coconut oil and the flax seed gel, mixing well to combine evenly.

5 In another bowl, stir together the chickpea flour, sesame seeds, coriander, cumin, chilli (if using) and Parmesan.

6 Pour the dry ingredients into the wet ingredients and mix together until well combined. Transfer the mixture to the prepared loaf tin, smoothing down with a spoon. Press the pepitas onto the top.

7 Bake in the oven for 40–45 minutes, or until an inserted skewer comes out clean. Remove from the oven and transfer to a wire rack in its baking paper lining. Remove the paper and return the loaf to the oven for a further 10 minutes, to brown up the sides.

8 Remove from the oven and allow to cool before slicing. Keep stored in the fridge for up to one week, slicing as needed.

MAKES 6–8 SLICES

This recipe
looks complex
but **trust us,**
it's *delicious!*

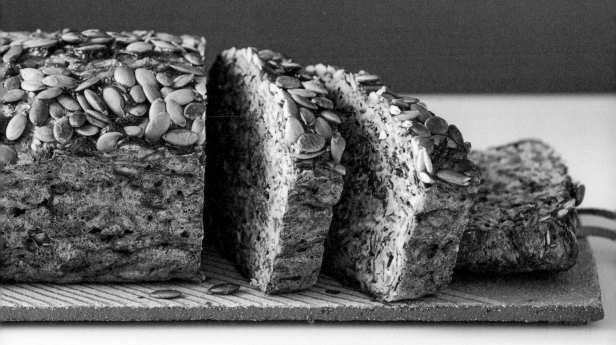

Homemade Sushi

Beautiful

5 nori sheets
1 cucumber
1 carrot

Unstoppable

300 g wild-caught salmon
(tinned or cooked), chopped
into small chunks

Fearless

1 avocado

DIPPING SAUCE
⅓ cup tamari
¼ cup white wine vinegar
1 teaspoon grated fresh ginger
½ teaspoon sesame oil

1. Chop thin, lengthways slices of cucumber, carrot and avocado.

2. Place the shiny side of the nori sheet down, narrow side towards you, and add pieces of salmon, cucumber, carrot and avocado on the two-thirds closest to you.

3. Carefully roll the nori sheet into a roll, sealing it by dabbing a bit of water along the top edge.

4. Using a sharp, serrated knife, cut the roll into several sections of desired thickness.

5. Combine the Dipping Sauce ingredients and serve alongside your sushi.

SERVES 2–3

Vegan option

REPLACE THE SALMON WITH MORE VEGETABLES, LIKE CAPSICUM, SPROUTS, PICKLES AND BEETROOT. VEGANS COULD ALSO ADD SOME COOKED BROWN RICE TO MAKE THEIR ROLLS A LITTLE MORE SUBSTANTIAL.

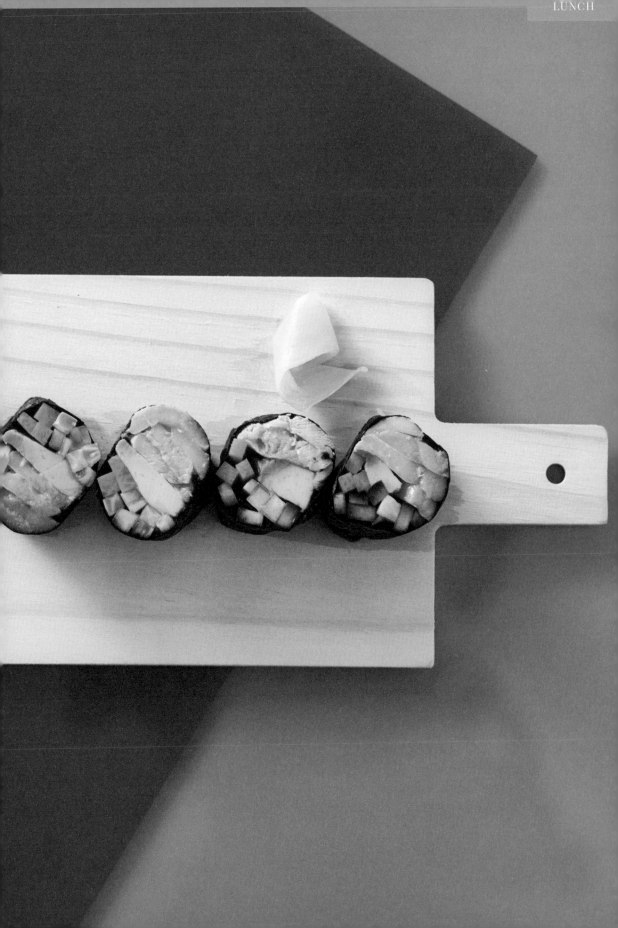

Brown Rice Poke Bowl

Beautiful

2 cups leafy greens (e.g. spinach,
rocket, cos lettuce)
1 Lebanese cucumber, thinly sliced
½ cup roughly chopped coriander
lemon wedges, to serve

Unstoppable

½ cup brown rice (to yield 1½ cups
cooked rice)
serve of tempeh, smoked salmon,
boiled eggs or poached chicken
2 tablespoons black sesame seeds

Fearless

½ avocado
sea salt and pepper, to taste

POKE DRESSING
2 tablespoons tahini
1 tablespoon tamari
1 tablespoon maple syrup
juice of ½ lemon

1 Place the rice and 1½ cups of water in a
saucepan, bring to the boil then simmer for
30 minutes. You may need to add a dash more
water in the cooking process.

2 Prepare your protein of choice.

3 To make the Poke Dressing, combine all the
dressing ingredients in a bowl and whisk well.

4 Construct the poke bowl by arranging the leafy
greens, cucumber, rice, avocado and protein of
choice in a bowl. Season with salt and pepper.
Top with coriander, a drizzle of Poke Dressing
and the sesame seeds and serve with lemon
wedges.

SERVES 2

Buf Girls' Tip

INSTEAD OF USING BROWN RICE,
YOU CAN USE ANY LEFTOVER GRAINS
OF YOUR CHOICE. VEGANS CAN REPLACE
THE SALMON AND EGG FOR MORE VEGGIES,
EXTRA AVOCADO OR BIG SCOOPS OF
HUMMUS WITH TOASTED SEEDS ON TOP.

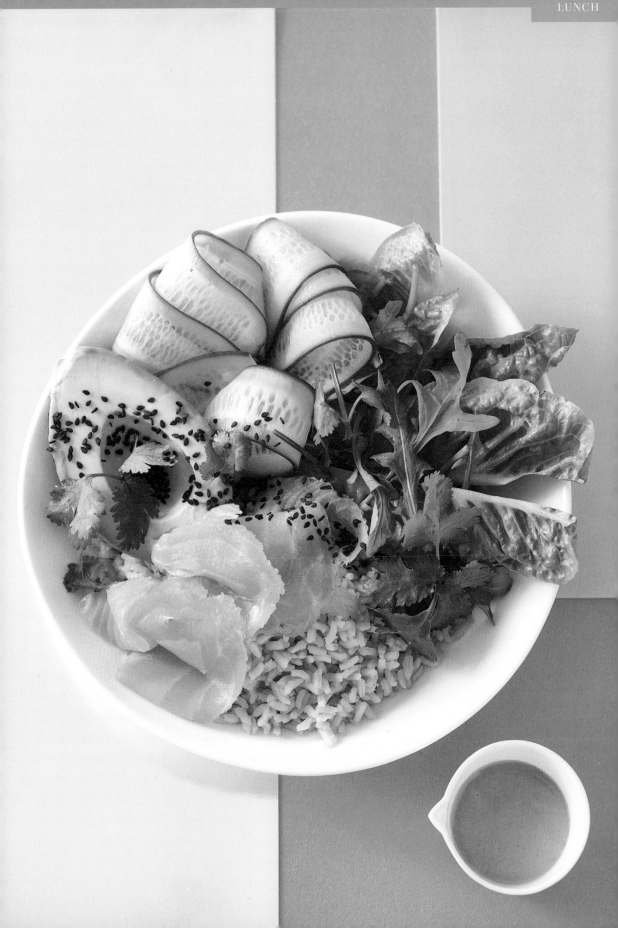

Cauli-fried Rice with Chicken

Beautiful

½ head of cauliflower, trimmed
    and cut into florets
1 zucchini, cut into chunks
1 clove garlic, crushed
1 small chilli, finely chopped
1 tablespoon grated fresh ginger
½ cup peas, fresh or frozen
½ cup roughly chopped coriander,
    to serve

Unstoppable

200 g chicken breast, cut into
    small pieces
¼ cup roughly chopped roasted
    cashews, to serve

Fearless

1 tablespoon coconut oil
1 teaspoon ground cumin
¼ cup water
2 tablespoons tamari

1   In a food processor, whiz the cauliflower and
zucchini until it resembles rice.

2   Place a frying pan over medium heat, add the
oil and fry the garlic, chilli, ginger and cumin for
2 minutes, then add the chicken and cook for
7–10 minutes, until the chicken is browned and
almost cooked through.

3   Next, add the cauliflower and zucchini 'rice'
with ¼ cup of water. Cook for 5 minutes, stirring,
then add the tamari and peas. Cook for a further
10 minutes, ideally covered with a lid to allow
the vegetables to steam and cook.

4   Dish up and top with coriander and cashews.

SERVES 2

Vegan option

REPLACE THE CHICKEN WITH
TEMPEH, TOFU, COOKED
LENTILS OR QUINOA.

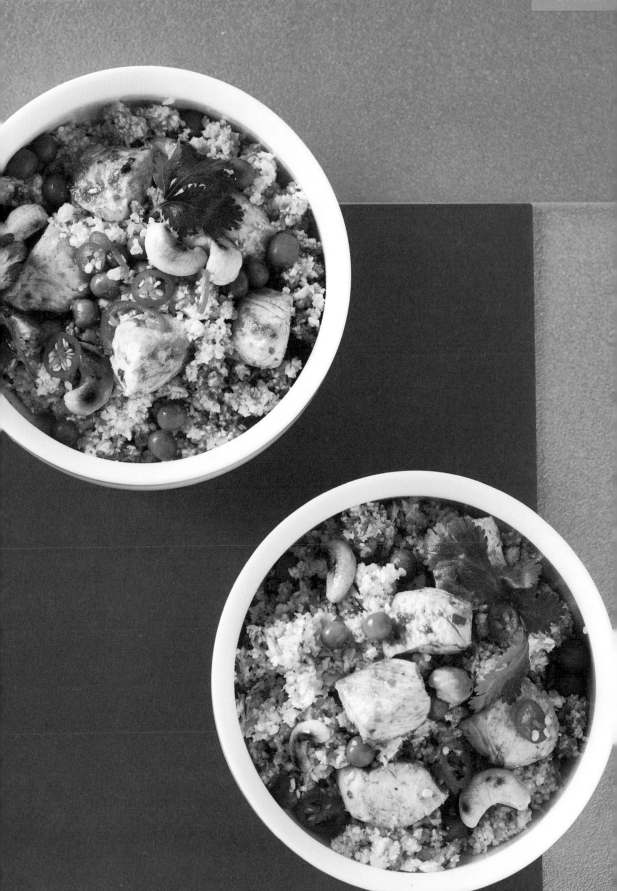

Cheeseburger with Carrot Fries

Beautiful

½ red onion, finely diced
¼ cup roughly chopped coriander
2 carrots, cut into chip-sized
    pieces
2 cups rocket
2 tomatoes, sliced

Unstoppable

500 g beef mince
1 egg
4 bread rolls (or lettuce leaves if
    you want a low-carb option)
4 slices tasty cheese of your choice

Fearless

2 tablespoons wholegrain mustard
1 tablespoon olive oil
sea salt and pepper, to taste
1 teaspoon paprika
1 avocado, mashed

YOGHURT DIJON SAUCE
    ½ cup natural yoghurt
    1 tablespoon Dijon mustard

1 Preheat the oven to 180°C and line two trays with baking paper.

2 In a bowl, combine the beef mince, egg, mustard, onion and coriander. Mix well, then form into four patties, molding firmly with your hands. Place on one of the baking trays and cook in the oven for 15–20 minutes, until the patties are cooked through.

3 In a bowl, toss the carrots with the olive oil, salt and pepper and paprika. Place on the second baking tray and cook for 15 minutes, or until the carrots are golden brown.

4 To make the Yoghurt Dijon Sauce, simply mix the yoghurt with the mustard.

5 To construct the burger, spread the avocado on the bread roll/lettuce leaf, then place the rocket, tomato, beef patty and cheese on top, finishing with the sauce.

> SERVES 4

Vegan option

REPLACE THE BEEF PATTIES
WITH ROAST VEGGIE PATTIES
(SEE RECIPE PAGE 170).

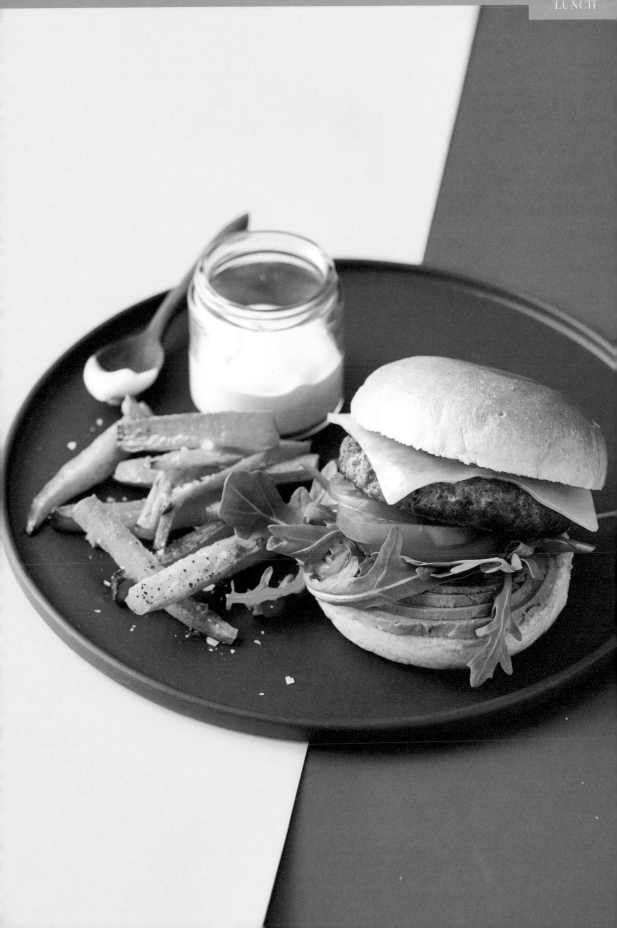

Chicken, Haloumi and Beetroot Salad

Beautiful

2 small beetroots, peeled and
    cut into quarters
1 cup spinach leaves

Unstoppable

150 g chicken breast, sliced
50 g haloumi, sliced

Fearless

1 tablespoon olive oil
sea salt and pepper, to taste

DRESSING
1 teaspoon wholegrain mustard
1 teaspoon honey
1 teaspoon water
juice of ½ lemon

1   Preheat the oven to 180°C and line a tray with baking paper.

2   In a bowl, toss together the beetroot, chicken and olive oil, and season with salt and pepper.

3   Place chicken and beetroot mixture on the baking tray and bake for 20 minutes, or until the chicken is cooked through and the beetroot is tender.

4   While the chicken is cooking, place a frying pan over medium heat and cook the haloumi for 2 minutes each side, or until golden.

5   To make the Dressing, simply combine all dressing ingredients in a bowl and mix well.

6   Once cooked, toss the chicken, beetroot, haloumi, spinach and dressing together. Serve immediately.

SERVES 1

Vegan option

REPLACE THE CHICKEN AND
HALOUMI WITH AVOCADO
AND WALNUTS, AND THE
HONEY WITH MAPLE SYRUP.

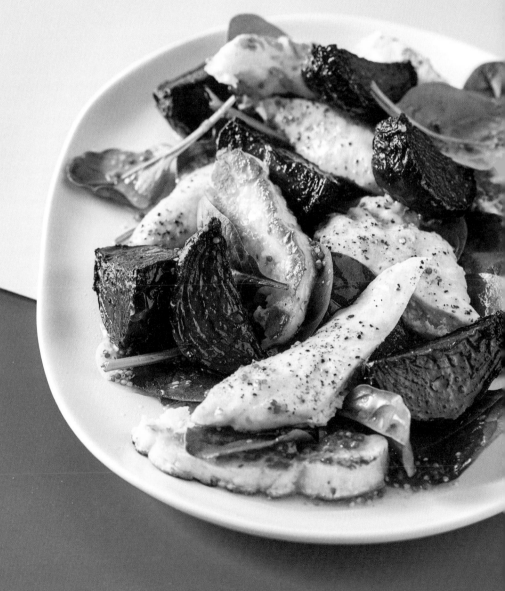

Coconut Poached Chicken with Leafy Greens

Beautiful

1 tablespoon grated fresh ginger
zest and juice of 1 lemon
2 cups spinach leaves or rocket
½ cup herbs of your choice
    (e.g. mint, coriander or Thai basil)

Unstoppable

1 chicken breast, cut in half
¼ cup crushed roasted cashews

Fearless

400 ml coconut milk
1 teaspoon ground cinnamon
sea salt and pepper, to taste

1   Place the chicken, coconut milk, ginger, cinnamon, lemon zest and salt and pepper in a saucepan and bring to a simmer. Cook for 15-20 minutes, or until the chicken is cooked all the way through.

2   Remove the chicken breast and shred with a fork.

3   Toss the green leaves with the herbs.

4   Serve the chicken over the salad and top with cashews and the lemon juice.

SERVES 2

Vegan option

SWAP THE CHICKEN BREAST FOR AN ORGANIC TOFU STEAK, OR A LARGE PORTOBELLO MUSHROOM.

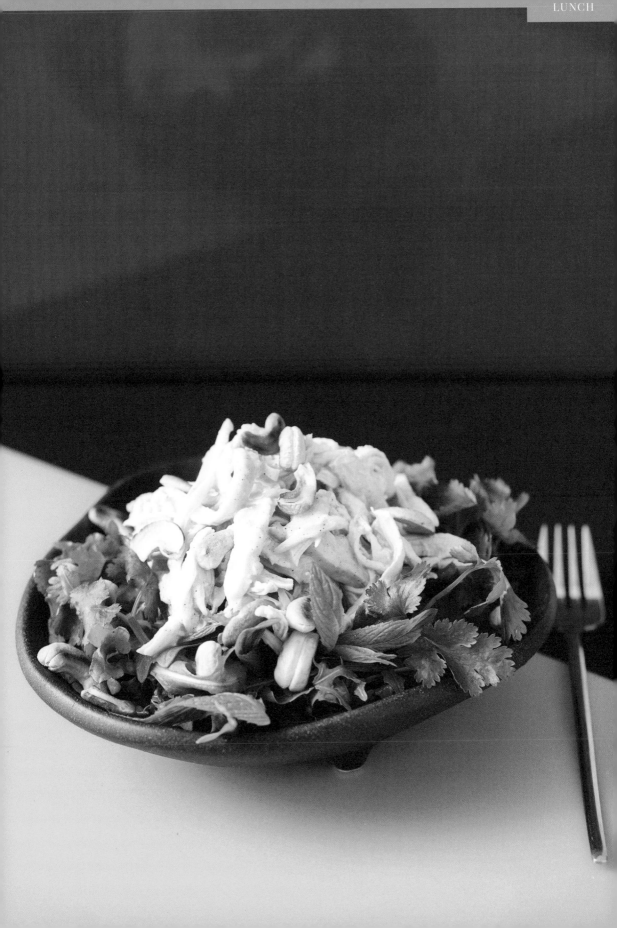

Crispy Chicken Salad

Beautiful

zest and juice of 1 lemon
500 g pumpkin, cut into small cubes
2 cups leafy greens (e.g. spinach,
   rocket, cos lettuce)

Unstoppable

¼ cup almond meal (or hazelnut
   meal for a different taste)
1 egg
1 chicken breast, thinly sliced

Fearless

¼ cup desiccated coconut
1 tablespoon chia seeds
2 tablespoons olive oil
sea salt and pepper, to taste

DRESSING
1 tablespoon olive oil
1 tablespoon tamari
1 tablespoon apple cider vinegar

1 Preheat the oven to 180°C and line a tray with baking paper.

2 Combine the almond meal, coconut, chia seeds and lemon zest in a bowl.

3 In a separate bowl, whisk the egg.

4 Coat the chicken in the egg, then coat the chicken in the almond meal mixture.

5 Heat a frying pan with 1 tablespoon of the olive oil and cook the chicken for 5–10 minutes, or until cooked and crispy.

6 Toss the pumpkin with the remaining olive oil and season with salt and pepper. Bake in the oven for 15 minutes, or until the pumpkin is tender. Allow to cool slightly.

7 Toss the leafy greens with the roasted pumpkin pieces.

8 To make the Dressing, combine the olive oil, tamari and apple cider vinegar. Toss through the salad and serve with the chicken.

SERVES 2

Vegan option

SUBSTITUTE THE CHICKEN FOR CHUNKS OF RYE BREAD, BROKEN UP AND FRIED IN YOUR PAN.

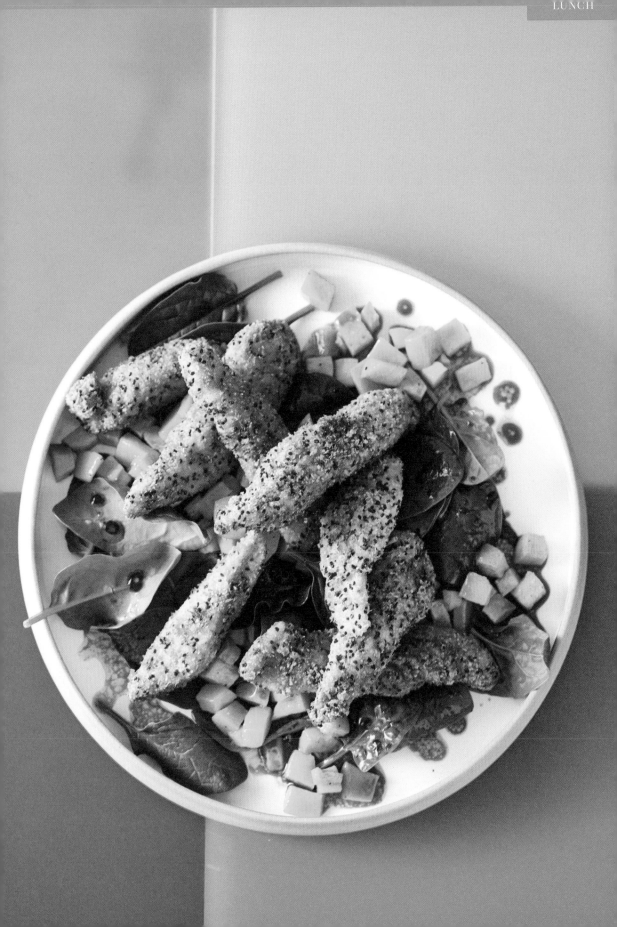

Apple and Haloumi Salad

Beautiful
1 red apple or 1 pear, cored and thinly sliced
1 cos lettuce, roughly chopped
zest and juice of 1 lemon

Unstoppable
200 g haloumi, sliced (or sliced firm tofu)

Fearless
¼ cup roughly chopped roasted almonds
1 tablespoon olive oil
1 tablespoon balsamic vinegar

1. Place a frying pan over medium heat and cook the haloumi slices for 2 minutes each side, or until golden. Remove the haloumi and cook the apple or pear for 2 minutes each side.
2. In a large bowl, toss together the lettuce, apple/ pear, haloumi, lemon zest and juice and roasted almonds. Drizzle over the olive oil and balsamic vinegar and serve.

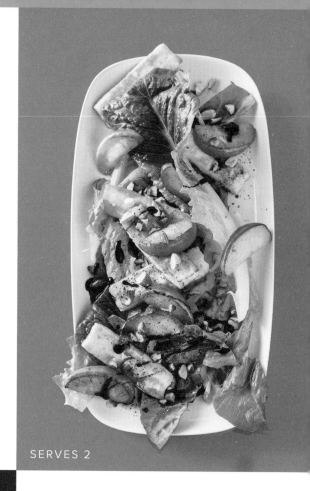

SERVES 2

Vegan option

LEAVE OUT THE GOAT'S FETA
AND ADD A FEW PECANS INSTEAD.

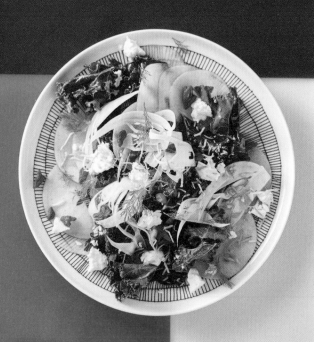

SERVES 2

Kale, Fennel and Apple Sala

Beautiful
4 cups roughly chopped kale
½ fennel bulb, thinly sliced
½ lemon

Unstoppable
1 red apple, cored and chopped into small pieces
2 tablespoons crumbled goat's feta
2 tablespoons goji berries

Fearless
¼ cup shredded coconut
1 tablespoon olive oil
½ teaspoon sea salt

1. Heat a small frying pan over medium heat and dry-fry the coconut. Remove and set aside.
2. Put the kale in a large bowl, add the olive oil and sa and gently massage the kale. Add the fennel, apple feta, goji berries and toasted coconut to the bowl and toss to combine.
3. To finish, squeeze over the juice of ½ lemon.

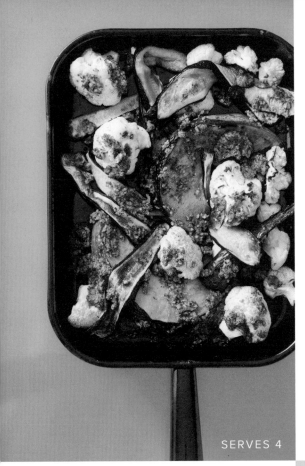

SERVES 4

Pesto Roast Vegetables

Beautiful
600 g pumpkin, sliced into wedges
½ cauliflower, cut into florets
2 zucchini, sliced into thick ribbons
Rocket Pesto (see recipe page 243)

1 Preheat the oven to 180°C and line a tray with baking paper.
2 In a bowl, toss the vegetables in the pesto, ensuring they are well coated. Transfer the vegetables to the tray and cook for 25 minutes, or until tender.

SERVES 2

Quinoa Bake

Beautiful
1 cup spinach leaves, roughly chopped
1 cup diced cooked vegetables of your choice, ideally leftovers (e.g. pumpkin, sweet potato, broccoli)

Unstoppable
½–1 cup cooked quinoa
4 eggs, lightly beaten (or vegan egg substitute)

Fearless
1 teaspoon chilli flakes (optional)
sea salt and pepper, to taste

Preheat the oven to 180°C and line a baking dish or tin with baking paper.

Mix all the ingredients together in a bowl, including chilli flakes if you like. Spoon into the prepared dish or tin and bake for 20–25 minutes, or until the egg is completely cooked.

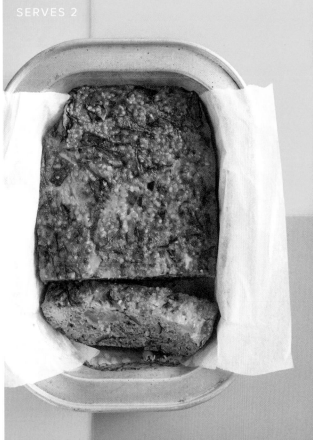

Mixed Roast Veg with Chicken

Beautiful

1 parsnip, cut into chunks
½ eggplant, cut into chunks
1 zucchini, cut into chunks
½ red onion, cut into chunks
2 cups spinach leaves
juice and zest of 1 lemon
½ cup roughly chopped coriander

Unstoppable

200 g chicken breast, cut into
    small pieces

Fearless

2 tablespoons olive oil
2 tablespoons balsamic vinegar
sea salt and pepper, to taste

1   Preheat the oven to 180°C and line a tray with
    baking paper.

2   In a large bowl, toss together the chicken,
    parsnip, eggplant, zucchini and red onion with
    the olive oil, 1 tablespoon of the balsamic
    vinegar, the lemon zest and salt and pepper.

3   Spread the vegetables and chicken onto the
    baking tray and bake for 25 minutes, or until
    golden brown and the chicken is cooked
    through.

4   Toss the cooked vegetables and chicken
    through the spinach and coriander and drizzle
    with lemon juice and the remaining balsamic
    vinegar.

SERVES 2

Vegan option

LEAVE OUT THE CHICKEN
AND ADD MORE VEGETABLES
FOR A ROAST VEGETABLE
SALAD OPTION.

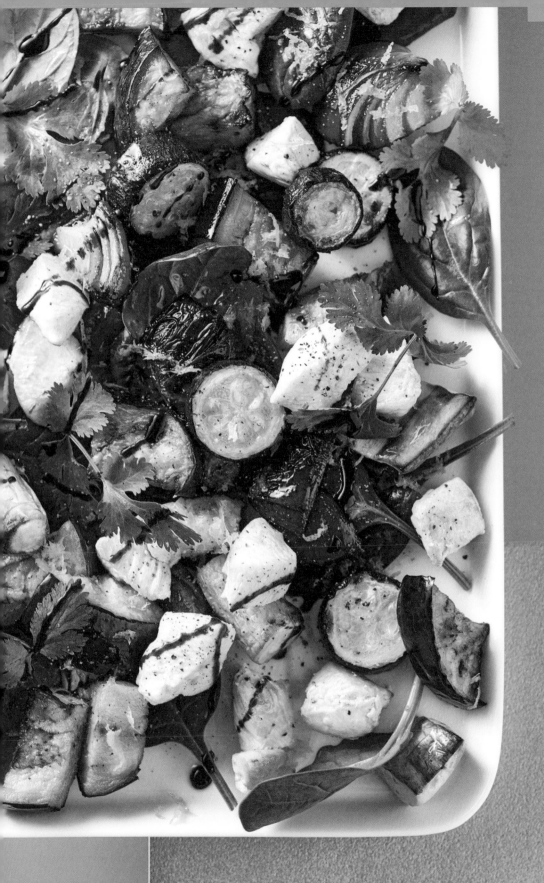

Mushroom and Tuna Bake

Beautiful

1 celery stick, chopped
1 tomato, chopped
2–3 portobello mushrooms, stalks
  removed
Italian parsley, chopped (a few
  leaves will do)

Unstoppable

90 g can tuna, in brine
sprinkle of Parmesan (optional)

Fearless

olive oil, for drizzling
spices (e.g. turmeric and paprika),
  to taste
sea salt and pepper, to taste

1 Preheat the oven to 180°C.

2 Combine the celery, tomato, tuna and Parmesan
   in a bowl. Add the spices and salt and pepper to
   suit your taste.

3 Place the mushrooms in an oven-safe dish,
   undersides upwards. Divide the tuna mix between
   your mushrooms, spooning into the cups.

4 Bake for 10 minutes. Remove from the oven and
   drizzle with a little olive oil before baking for
   another 5 minutes.

5 Remove from the oven, sprinkle with parsley and
   cover with aluminium foil for about 5 minutes.

6 Remove foil and serve.

SERVES 1

Buf Girls' Tip

THIS IS FANTASTIC TO EAT
ON ITS OWN, OR ALONGSIDE
A BIG SERVE OF GREEN
VEGETABLES AND A LITTLE
BROWN RICE.

Vegan option

SIMPLY FILL THE
MUSHROOM CUPS WITH
MORE VEGETABLES.

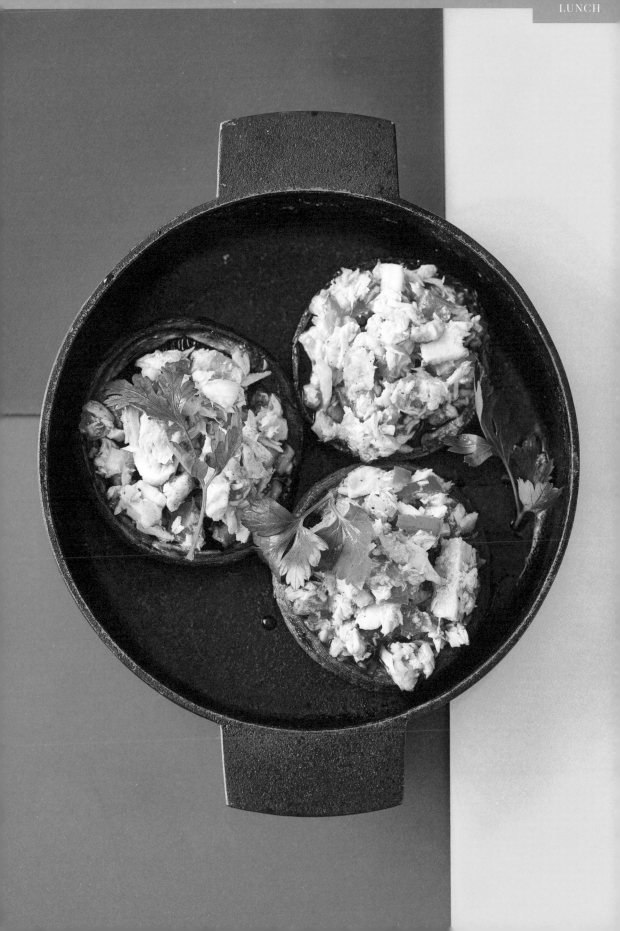

Open Chicken Sanga

Beautiful

2 cos lettuce leaves
1 tomato, sliced
1 handful of alfalfa

Unstoppable

150 g chicken breast (about half
  a small chicken breast)
1 slice of bread
1 tablespoon hummus or Avocado
  and Chickpea Hummus
  (see recipe page 243)

Fearless

½ tablespoon olive oil
1 tablespoon finely chopped fresh
  oregano
sea salt and pepper, to taste
1 tablespoon Fresh Pesto (see
  recipe page 247)
¼–½ avocado

1 Coat the chicken breast with olive oil and
   season with oregano, salt and pepper. Place
   a frying pan over medium heat and cook the
   chicken for 7 minutes each side, or until the
   chicken is cooked through. Allow to cool a little.

2 Construct your sandwich by spreading pesto
   onto the bread, then top with hummus, lettuce,
   tomato, chicken, avocado and alfalfa.

SERVES 1

Vegan option

REPLACE THE CHICKEN
WITH EXTRA AVOCADO OR
YOUR CHOICE OF SALAD
VEGETABLE.

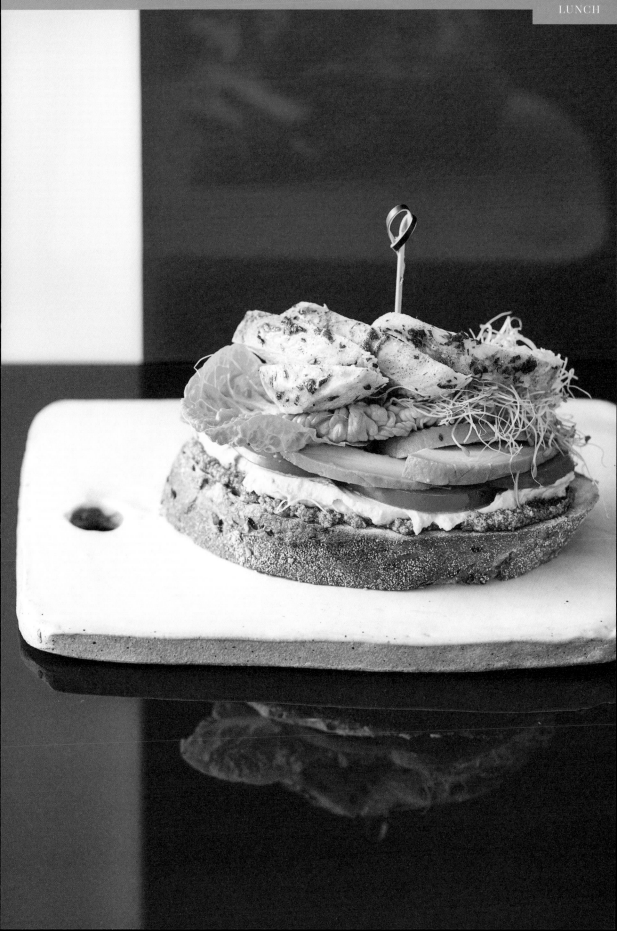

Pearl Barley and Bean Salad

Beautiful

2 cups rocket

1 cup green beans, topped and
tailed and cut in half

½ cup pearl barley (yields 1½ cups
of cooked barley)

Unstoppable

200 g (½ can) four-bean mix,
drained and rinsed

Fearless

sea salt and pepper, to taste

DRESSING

juice of ½ lemon

1 tablespoon olive oil

1 tablespoon wholegrain mustard

1 tablespoon balsamic vinegar

1   To cook the barley, place the barley and 1½ cups
of water in a saucepan, bring to the boil then
simmer for 30 minutes. You may need to add a
dash more water in the cooking process.

2   In a bowl, combine the rocket, green beans,
four-bean mix and cooked barley.

3   Combine all the Dressing ingredients in a small
bowl and mix well.

4   Pour dressing over the salad, season with salt
and pepper, and serve.

SERVES 2

Buf Girls' Tip

SERVE WITH AN EXTRA
PORTION OF PROTEIN
(E.G. CHICKEN, EGGS,
BEEF OR TEMPEH).

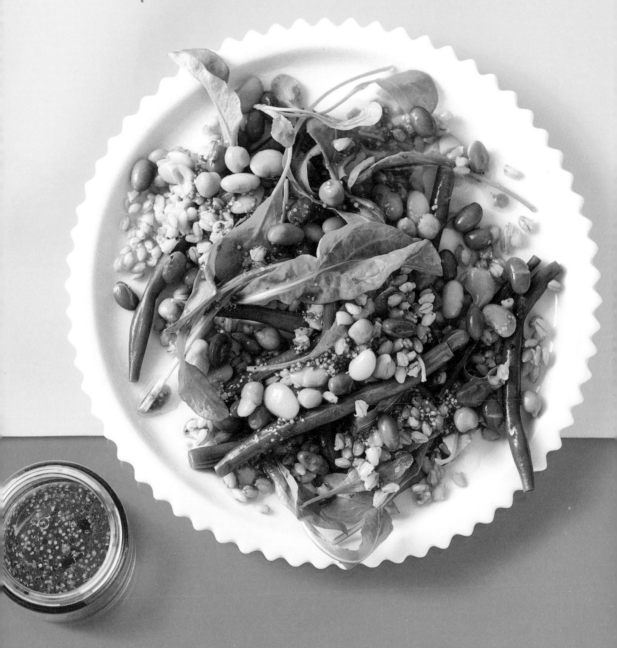

'Buf Girls'
post-training fave!

Pho Bowl

Beautiful

1 tablespoon grated fresh ginger
2 carrots, thinly sliced
2 cups wombok cabbage (or any
    cabbage), thinly sliced
2 zucchini, spiralised
1 cup bean sprouts
1 handful of mint leaves, to serve
1 lime, to serve

Unstoppable

2 chicken breasts, thinly sliced

Fearless

1 litre vegetable broth or salt-
    reduced stock
2 cups water
2 star anise (optional)
1 cinnamon stick
½ teaspoon chilli powder
1 teaspoon sea salt

1   In a large saucepan, combine the broth, water, star anise, cinnamon stick, chilli powder, salt and ginger. Bring to the boil, add the sliced chicken, then reduce heat to a simmer. Simmer for 15 minutes, or until the chicken is cooked through. Remove the star anise and cinnamon stick.

2   Place the carrot and cabbage into the saucepan and cook for another 5 minutes, or until the carrot is tender. Turn off the heat.

3   Prepare four large bowls to dish up the pho.

4   Divide the spiralised zucchini noodles between the bowls, then add a generous scoop of the broth mixture.

5   To serve, top with the bean sprouts, mint leaves and a squeeze of lime juice.

SERVES 4

Vegan option

REPLACE THE CHICKEN
WITH TOFU OR THIN SLICES
OF PUMPKIN.

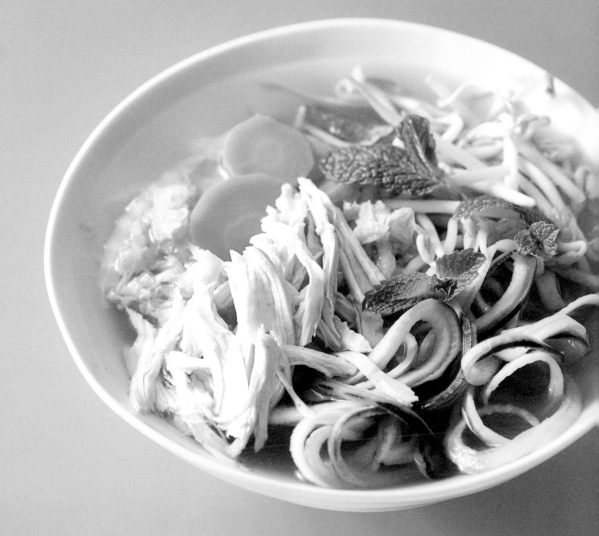

Pumpkin & Broccolini Salad with Walnuts

Beautiful

1 bunch of broccolini, trimmed
   and cut in half
500 g pumpkin, cut into cubes
1 cup spinach leaves
½ lemon

Unstoppable

½ cup quinoa (yields 1½ cups
   of cooked quinoa)

Fearless

2 tablespoons olive oil
1 teaspoon cinnamon
½ teaspoon salt
¼ cup roughly chopped walnuts
1 tablespoon apple cider vinegar
sea salt and pepper, to taste

1   Preheat the oven to 180°C and line a tray with baking paper.

2   In a bowl, toss the pumpkin cubes with 1 tablespoon of the olive oil, plus the cinnamon and salt. Tip the pumpkin onto the baking tray and bake for 15 minutes, or until tender.

3   While the pumpkin is cooking, cook the quinoa by adding 1 cup of water to the quinoa in a saucepan and bringing to the boil. Once boiling, turn the heat down to a simmer and cook with the lid on for 15 minutes, or until the water has been absorbed and the quinoa is cooked.

4   Place the broccolini in a heatproof bowl and pour freshly boiled water over the top. Allow the broccolini to blanch for 5 minutes, then drain. The stems should be tender.

5   In a large bowl, combine the spinach, cooked pumpkin, broccolini, quinoa and walnuts. Dress with apple cider vinegar, the remaining olive oil and a squeeze of lemon juice. Season with salt and pepper and it's ready to eat.

SERVES 2

Buf Girls' Tip

EXTRA HUNGRY, OR YOU'VE JUST WRAPPED UP A GIANT TRAINING SESSION? SERVE WITH AN EXTRA PORTION OF PROTEIN, SUCH AS CHICKEN, EGGS OR TEMPEH.

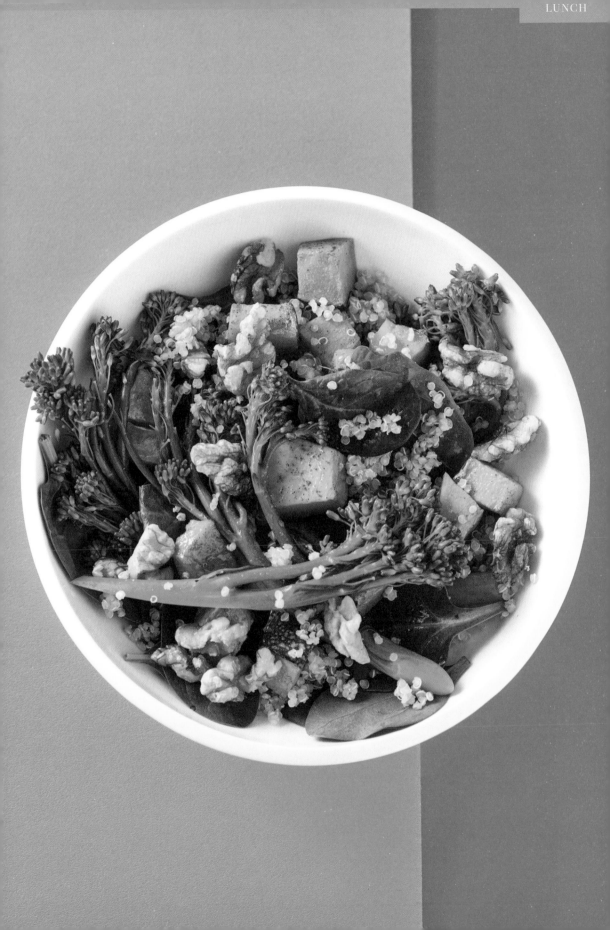

Rainbow Abundance Bowl

Beautiful

250 g pumpkin, cut into small
    cubes
2 cups rocket
1 capsicum, diced
8 cherry tomatoes, halved
1 Lebanese cucumber, diced
1 lemon

Unstoppable

200 g chicken breast, cut into
    small pieces
½ cup quinoa (yields 1½ cups
    of cooked quinoa)

Fearless

1 tablespoon olive oil
1 tablespoon cinnamon
½ teaspoon sea salt
½ avocado, sliced
1 tablespoon tahini
sea salt and pepper, to taste

1. Preheat the oven to 180°C and line a tray with baking paper.

2. In a bowl, toss the pumpkin cubes and chicken with the olive oil, cinnamon and salt.

3. Place the pumpkin and chicken on the tray and cook in the oven for 20 minutes, or until the chicken is cooked through.

4. To cook the quinoa, place in a saucepan, add 1 cup of water and bring to the boil. Once boiling, turn the heat down to a simmer and cook with the lid on for 15 minutes, or until the water has absorbed and quinoa is cooked.

5. Once all the cooked elements are complete, it's time to build your bowl. Arrange the rocket, capsicum, cherry tomatoes, cucumber, chicken, pumpkin, quinoa and avocado in your bowl. Finish with a drizzle of tahini, a squeeze of lemon juice, and season with salt and pepper.

SERVES 2

Vegan option

REPLACE THE CHICKEN
WITH ROAST VEGGIE PATTIES
(SEE RECIPE PAGE 170).

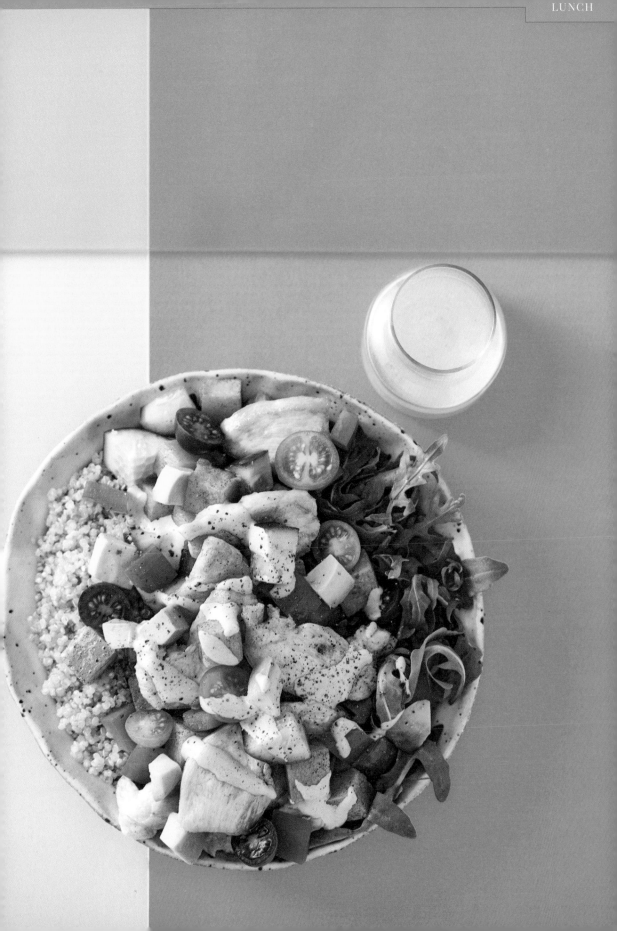

Raw Broccoli Salad with Curry Cashew Dressing

Beautiful

2 heads of broccoli
¼ cup goji berries

Unstoppable

¼ cup sunflower seeds

Fearless

¼ cup shredded coconut

CURRY CASHEW DRESSING
juice of ½ lemon
1 cup raw cashews, soaked for
    at least 4 hours or overnight
½ – ¾ cup water
2 teaspoons curry powder
1 teaspoon sea salt

1 Finely dice the broccoli and place in a large bowl.

2 Heat a small frying pan over medium heat and dry-fry the sunflower seeds and shredded coconut. Remove from the pan when lightly golden.

3 To make the Curry Cashew Dressing, drain the soaked cashews and place in a blender with the lemon juice, ½ cup water, curry powder and salt. Blend until the mixture is of a smooth consistency. Add more water if the dressing seems too thick.

4 Pour dressing into the bowl with the broccoli and thoroughly coat the broccoli. Finally, toss in the toasted sunflower seeds, shredded coconut and goji berries and gently combine.

SERVES 4

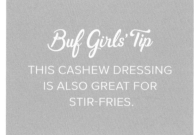

Buf Girls' Tip
THIS CASHEW DRESSING
IS ALSO GREAT FOR
STIR-FRIES.

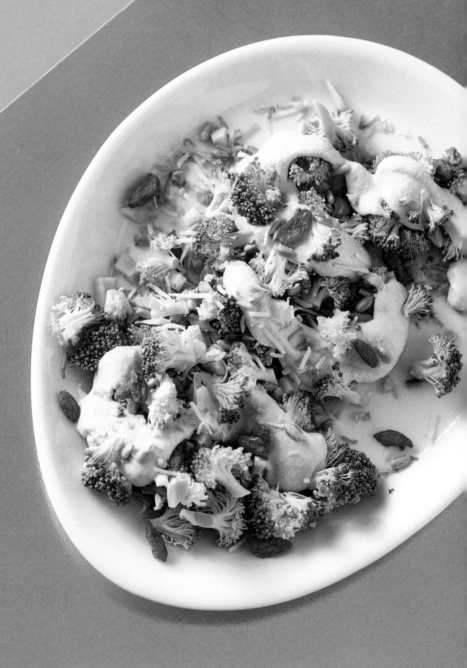

Roast Veggie Patties

Beautiful

300 g sweet potato, cut into small
  cubes
1 carrot, grated
½ cup finely chopped coriander

Unstoppable

400 g can lentils, drained and rinsed
1 egg, lightly beaten
⅓ cup coconut flour
2 tablespoons almond butter
2 tablespoons sunflower seeds

Fearless

2 teaspoons curry powder
1 tablespoon chia seeds
1 teaspoon sea salt

1 Preheat the oven to 180°C and line a tray with baking paper.

2 Place the sweet potato in a saucepan, cover with water and boil until soft. Drain and mash with a fork, then allow to cool slightly.

3 While the sweet potato is cooking, combine the carrot, coriander, lentils, egg, coconut flour, almond butter, curry powder, chia seeds and salt in a large bowl. Once the sweet potato is cooked and slightly cooled, add it to the mixture and combine well.

4 Form the mixture into 12 balls and place onto the prepared tray. Sprinkle the sunflower seeds over the patties and press down lightly to ensure the seeds stick.

5 Cook in the oven for 20 minutes, or until the patties are golden brown.

MAKES 12 PATTIES

Buf Girls' Tip

SERVE THE PATTIES WITH YOUR SALAD OF CHOICE, FOR EXAMPLE GRATED SALAD WITH TAHINI DRESSING (SEE RECIPE PAGE 134), OR TOP WITH SOME SMASHED AVOCADO OR AVOCADO AND CHICKPEA HUMMUS (SEE RECIPE PAGE 243).

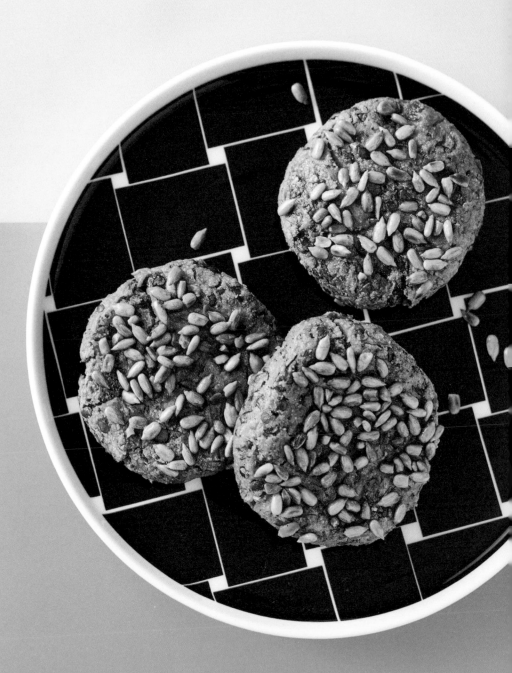

Spiced Beef Mince with Kimchi

Beautiful

1 clove garlic, crushed
1 small red chilli, finely chopped
1 head of broccoli, cut into florets
2 cups finely shredded red cabbage
2 cups spinach leaves

Unstoppable

500 g beef mince
¼ cup nuts and seeds of your
   choice

Fearless

1 tablespoon olive oil
4 tablespoons kimchi
1 avocado, sliced

1   Place a frying pan over medium-high heat, add the olive oil and sauté the garlic and chilli for 2 minutes, or until fragrant. Add the beef mince, stirring until browned. Add the chopped broccoli and cook for a further 5 minutes, until the mince is fully cooked and the broccoli is tender.

2   In a bowl, toss the cabbage with the kimchi.

3   Serve the mince and broccoli with the cabbage and kimchi mix, spinach and avocado. Top with nuts and seeds.

SERVES 4

Vegan option

SWAP THE MINCE FOR
1 CUP OF BLACK BEANS
AND 1 CUP OF COOKED
BROWN RICE.

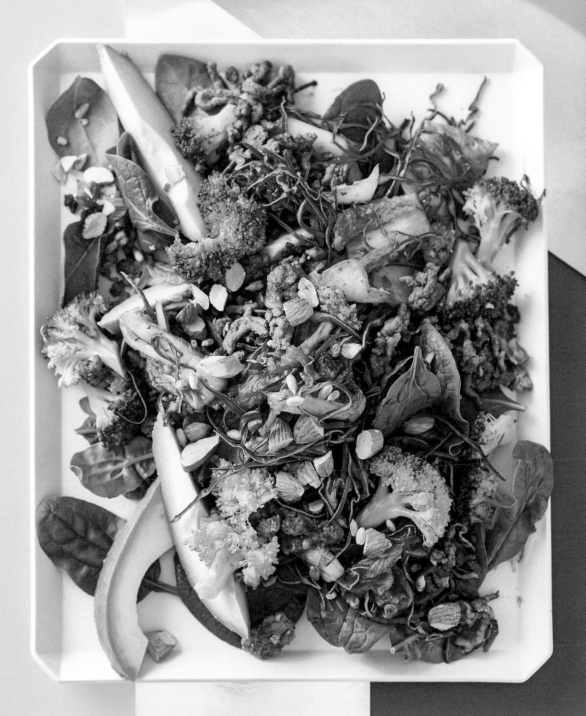

Triple C Patties with Asian Slaw

Beautiful

½ cup roughly chopped coriander

Unstoppable

1 egg, lightly beaten
500 g chicken mince
1 tablespoon tapioca flour
¼ cup LSA

Fearless

1 teaspoon ground cumin
1 teaspoon sea salt

ASIAN SLAW

2 carrots, spiralised
½ cup roughly chopped coriander
100 g snow peas, topped and tailed
    and thinly sliced
¼ small wombok cabbage, finely
    shredded

SLAW DRESSING

1 tablespoon grated fresh ginger
2 teaspoons honey or maple syrup
1 tablespoon olive oil
2 tablespoons tamari

1. Preheat the oven to 180°C and line a tray with baking paper.

2. Place all ingredients for the patties in a large bowl and mix until well combined. Form into patties.

3. Place the patties on the tray and bake for 20 minutes, or until the chicken is cooked and the patties start to turn golden brown.

4. While the patties are cooking, prepare the Asian Slaw.

5. In a bowl, mix together all the dressing ingredients and set aside.

6. In a separate, larger bowl, mix together the carrots, coriander, snow peas and cabbage.

7. Toss the dressing through the salad. Serve patties with the Asian Slaw.

SERVES 2

Vegan option

REPLACE THE CHICKEN WITH A MIX OF 1 CUP OF CANNED CANNELLINI OR KIDNEY BEANS AND 1 CUP OF DICED FIRM TOFU, AND REPLACE THE EGG WITH ½ CUP OF MASHED SWEET POTATO AND ½ CUP OF DESICCATED COCONUT.

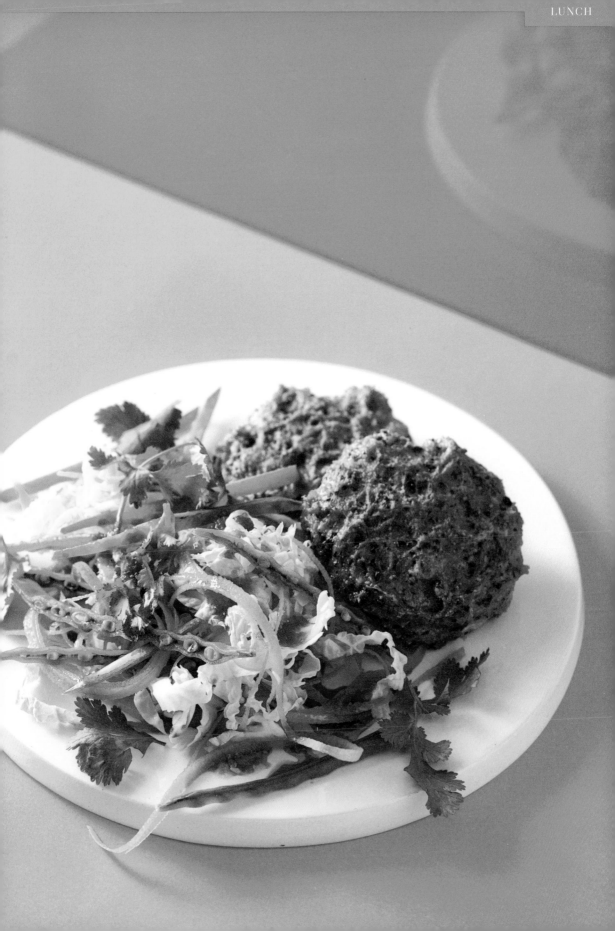

Zucchini and Turmeric Soup

Beautiful

1 red onion, roughly chopped
2 cloves garlic, crushed
6 zucchini, roughly chopped

Unstoppable

1 cup coconut milk

Fearless

1 tablespoon olive oil
4 teaspoons ground turmeric
2 teaspoons curry powder
1 teaspoon sea salt
6 cups (1.5 litres) vegetable stock
sea salt and pepper, to taste

1   Place a large saucepan over medium heat, add the olive oil and sauté the onion and garlic for 5 minutes, or until the onion becomes translucent. Add the turmeric, curry powder and 1 teaspoon of salt and stir for 3 minutes to let the flavours release. Add the vegetable stock, coconut milk and zucchini and simmer for 15 minutes, or until the zucchini is soft.

2   Allow to cool slightly, then transfer to a blender. Whiz to combine.

3   Return to the saucepan to reheat, season again with salt and pepper, if desired, and serve.

SERVES 4

Buf Girls' Tip

TO GET AN EXTRA PROTEIN BOOST YOU CAN ADD A SERVE OF SHREDDED CHICKEN BREAST, TEMPEH OR A BOILED EGG.

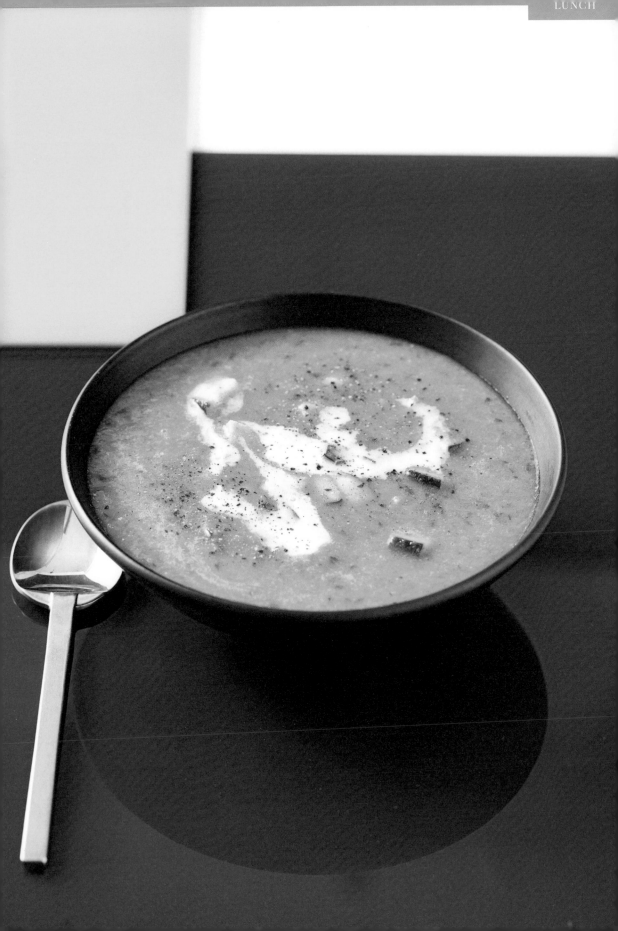

Baked Eggplant and Lentils

Beautiful

2 eggplants, cut in halves
   lengthways
400 g can crushed tomatoes
½ cup roughly chopped parsley
1 red onion, roughly chopped

Unstoppable

400 g can lentils, drained and
   rinsed
100 g goat's feta, crumbled

Fearless

3 tablespoons olive oil
sea salt, to taste
1 tablespoon balsamic vinegar
1 teaspoon ground cumin

1   Preheat the oven to 180°C and line a tray
    with baking paper.

2   In a bowl, coat the eggplant halves with
    2 tablespoons of the olive oil, and salt to taste.
    Place the eggplants flesh-side down on the tray
    and bake for 15 minutes, or until tender. Allow
    to cool slightly, then remove most of the flesh
    from the eggplants, leaving 1 cm of flesh around
    the skin. TIP: keep the flesh and add to your next
    lunch or dinner!

3   In a frying pan, heat the remaining olive oil and
    add the red onion. Cook, stirring, for 2 minutes,
    or until the onion starts to turn translucent.
    Add salt, balsamic vinegar and cumin and stir
    for another minute. Finally, add the tomatoes,
    parsley and lentils and cook for a further
    5 minutes.

4   Spoon the mixture into the hollowed-out
    eggplants and top with feta. Place the
    eggplants back into the oven for 5 minutes
    to melt the feta and heat through.

SERVES 2

Vegan option

JUST LEAVE OUT THE
FETA AND FOLLOW THE
REST OF THE RECIPE.

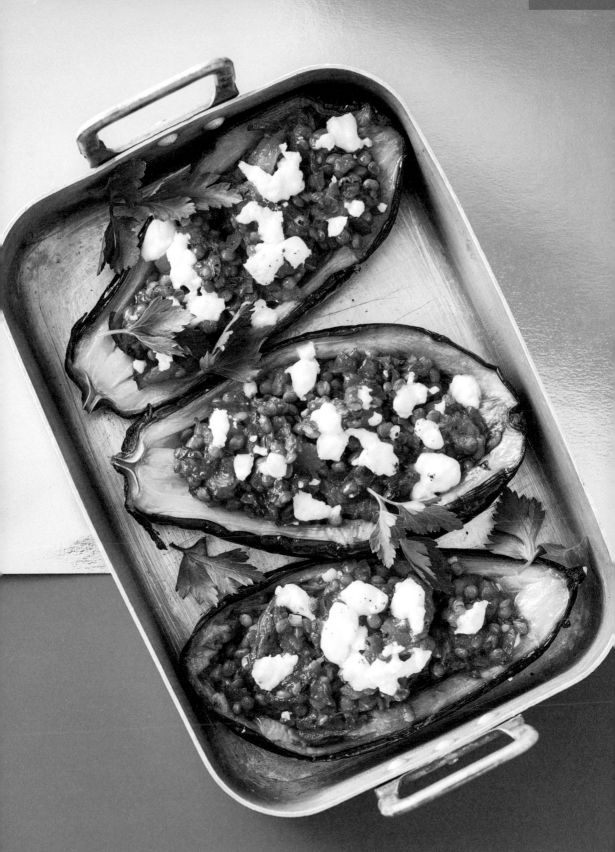

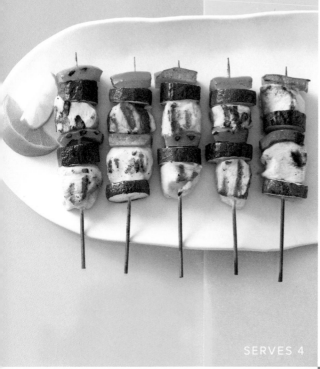

BBQ Chicken and Lime Skewers

Beautiful

1 red capsicum, deseeded and cut into 2 cm pieces
1 zucchini, cut into 2 cm cubes
1 clove garlic, crushed
2 limes

Unstoppable

2 chicken breasts, cut into cubes

Fearless

1 tablespoon olive oil

1. Juice 1 lime and add the juice to a bowl with the garlic, chicken and olive oil. Allow the chicken to marinate in the fridge for 20–30 minutes.
2. Thread chicken onto skewers, alternating with zucchini and capsicum chunks. Squeeze over the juice of the remaining lime.
3. Heat a large grill or frying pan over medium-high heat and cook the skewers for 8–10 minutes, turning often, until the chicken is cooked through.

SERVES 4

Broccoli, Goji and Avocado Salad

Beautiful

1 head of broccoli, cut into florets
¼ cup goji berries
2 cups rocket

Unstoppable

¼ cup roughly chopped roasted almonds

Fearless

1 avocado, quartered
1 serve Balsamic Vinaigrette
   (see recipe page 247)

1. Blanch the broccoli in boiling water for 3-5 minutes, or until tender.
2. In a large bowl, combine the broccoli, goji berries, rocket, roasted almonds and avocado.
3. Pour the Balsamic Vinaigrette dressing over the salad and toss to combine.

SERVES 2

Buf Girls' Tip
SERVE WITH YOUR CHOICE OF ADDED PROTEIN.

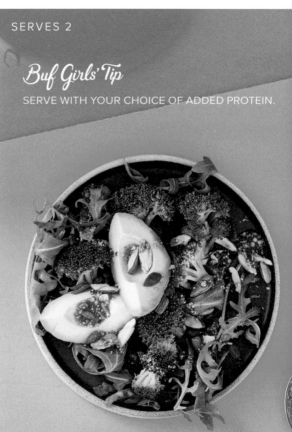

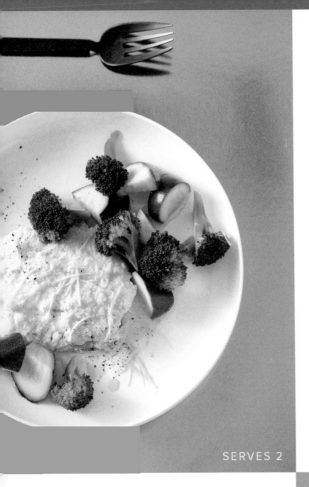

Ginger and Garlic Fish Parcels

Beautiful
2 tablespoons grated fresh ginger
2 cloves garlic, crushed
juice and zest of 1 lemon

Unstoppable
2 x fish fillets (e.g. snapper), about 150 g each
    (or 300g tempeh, sliced)

Fearless
2 tablespoons olive oil
sea salt and pepper, to taste

1 Preheat the oven to 180°C.
2 To prepare the dressing, mix together the ginger,
   garlic, lemon zest and olive oil.
3 Cut two large squares of aluminium foil and place
   a fish fillet on each. Pour over the dressing and
   season with salt and pepper. Fold the aluminium
   foil over to form parcels for the fish.
4 Place the fish parcels on an ovenproof tray and
   bake for 20 minutes, or until the fish is fully cooked
   through. To serve, drizzle over the lemon juice.

SERVES 2

SERVES 2

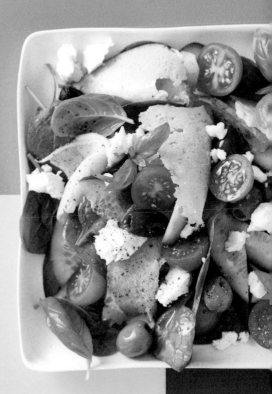

Mediterranean Salad

Beautiful
1 Lebanese cucumber, chopped into 2 cm pieces
1 punnet cherry tomatoes, halved
2 cups spinach leaves
½ cup olives
¼ cup roughly chopped basil
juice of 1 lemon

Unstoppable
150 g ham off the bone, torn into pieces (optional)
2 tablespoons goat's feta (or vegan feta), crumbled

Fearless
1 tablespoon olive oil
1 tablespoon apple cider vinegar
sea salt and pepper, to taste

1 Toss the cucumber, tomato, spinach, olives and
   basil together in a bowl.
2 To make the dressing, simply combine the lemon
   juice, olive oil and vinegar.
3 Toss the dressing through the salad, then top with
   ham and feta and season with salt and pepper.

Beef Satay Stir-fry

Beautiful

1 red capsicum, deseeded and
   thinly sliced
1 carrot, thinly sliced
100 g snow peas, topped and tailed
½ cup roughly chopped coriander,
   to serve

Unstoppable

500 g beef strips
1 cup quinoa (yields 3 cups of
   cooked quinoa)

Fearless

1 tablespoon olive oil

SATAY SAUCE
1 tablespoon grated fresh ginger
juice of ½ lemon
1 chilli, finely chopped
2 tablespoons maple syrup
3 tablespoons peanut butter
   (or almond butter)
1 tablespoon tamari
¼ cup water

1 To cook the quinoa, place the quinoa in a
   saucepan, add 3 cups of water and bring to
   the boil. Once boiling, turn the heat down to a
   simmer and cook with the lid on for 15 minutes,
   or until the water has been absorbed and the
   quinoa is cooked.

2 To make the Satay Sauce, mix all the sauce
   ingredients together in a jug and whisk well.

3 Place a frying pan over high heat, add the oil
   and cook the beef strips for 5 minutes, or until
   browned. Add the capsicum, carrot and snow
   peas and cook for 2 minutes, then mix in the
   satay sauce and cook for a further 5–7 minutes,
   until the vegetables are tender.

4 Serve the satay on a bed of quinoa and garnish
   with coriander.

SERVES 4

Vegan option

SUBSTITUTE TEMPEH
STRIPS, BLACK BEANS OR
NOODLES FOR THE MEAT.

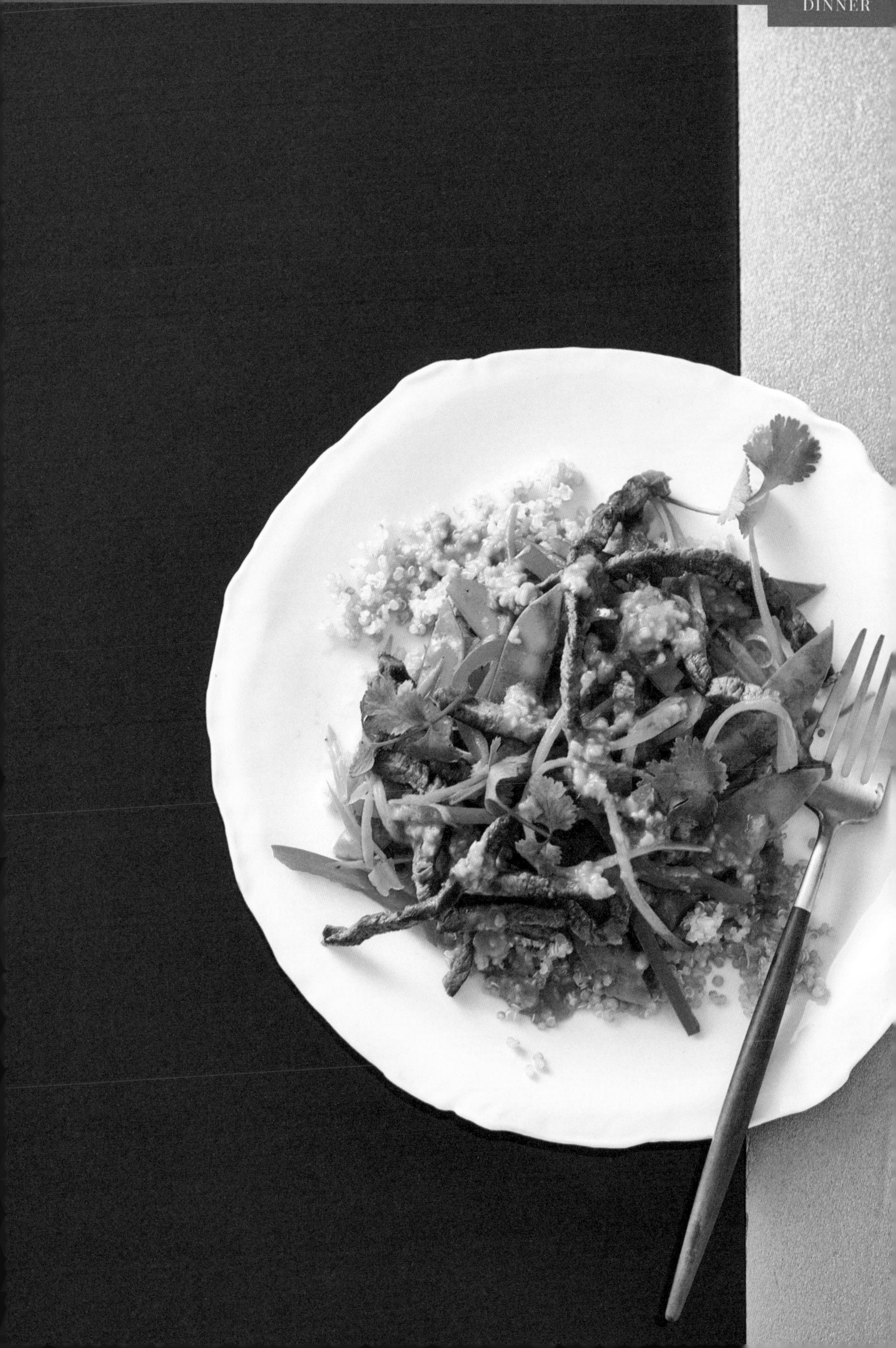

Brinner Frittata

Beautiful

3 zucchini, grated

2 carrots, grated

2 cups roughly chopped spinach leaves

8 cherry tomatoes, halved

Unstoppable

12 eggs (or vegan egg substitute)

¼ cup almond milk

100 g feta (or cubed tofu)

Fearless

sea salt and pepper, to taste

1 Preheat the oven to 170°C and line a square tin or frittata tray with baking paper.

2 In a large bowl, whisk the eggs and almond milk and season with salt and pepper.

3 Add in the grated zucchini, carrot and chopped spinach, and mix to combine.

4 Pour the egg and vegetable mixture into the tin. Arrange the cherry tomatoes and feta on top and bake for 30 minutes.

5 Remove from the oven and allow to cool for 2 minutes. Turn out onto a board and serve warm or at room temperature, sliced into squares.

SERVES 6

Buf Girls' Tip

YOU CAN ADD 2 CUPS OF ANY LEFTOVER ROAST VEG AS A REPLACEMENT FOR THE ZUCCHINI AND CARROTS.

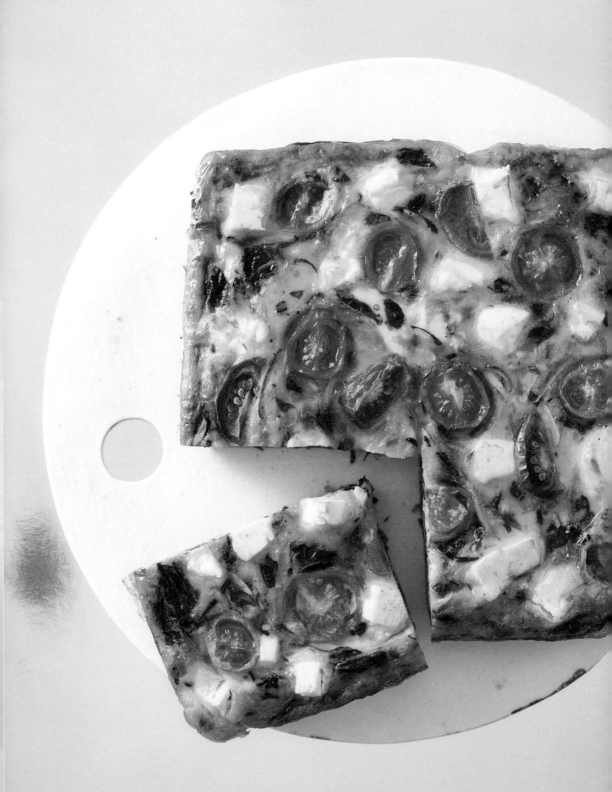

Cashew Butter Stir-fry

Beautiful

1 clove garlic, finely chopped
1 red chilli, chopped
2 cups chopped broccoli
2 cups chopped cauliflower
1 cup finely shredded cabbage

Unstoppable

400 g chicken breast, thinly sliced
¼ cup roughly chopped roasted
   cashews

Fearless

1 tablespoon olive oil
sea salt and pepper, to taste

CASHEW BUTTER SAUCE
⅓ cup cashew butter
2 tablespoons tamari
1 teaspoon apple cider vinegar
juice of ½ lemon
¼ cup water

1   To make the Cashew Butter Sauce, place all the sauce ingredients in a small bowl and mix until well combined.

2   Place a frying pan over medium-high heat, add the olive oil and cook the garlic and chilli for 2 minutes. Add the chicken strips and cook for a further 5 minutes. Add the broccoli, cauliflower and cabbage and cook, covered, for 5 minutes, or until the veggies begin to tenderise. Mix in the Cashew Butter Sauce and cook for a further 5 minutes.

3   Season with salt and pepper and serve sprinkled with the roasted cashews.

SERVES 4

Vegan option

REPLACE THE CHICKEN WITH NOODLES, RICE OR ADDITIONAL STARCHY VEGGIES, LIKE SWEET POTATO.

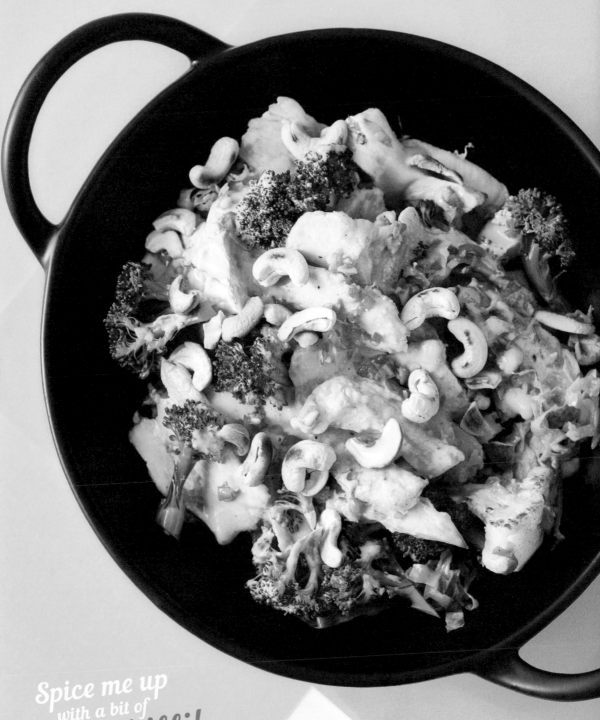

Spice me up
with a bit of
extra chilli!

Chicken Burgers with Sweet Potato Chips

Beautiful

1 small handful of mint, roughly
chopped
1 small handful of coriander,
roughly chopped

Unstoppable

500 g chicken mince
1 egg

Fearless

sea salt and pepper, to taste
2 tablespoons coconut oil
chilli flakes or cayenne pepper,
to taste

'BUNS' AND FILLINGS
cos or iceberg lettuce leaves
(as buns)
baby spinach leaves
sliced tomato
sliced avocado
goat's or sheep's feta, crumbled

SWEET POTATO CHIPS
1 large sweet potato
2 tablespoons coconut oil
spices (e.g. cinnamon,
cardamom, chilli)

1   Preheat the oven to 180°C.

2   In a bowl, mix together the chicken mince, egg,
mint, coriander and salt and pepper to taste.

3   Divide the mixture into eight patties and place
on a plate lined with baking paper. Refrigerate
for 30 minutes.

4   Meanwhile, wash and dry the sweet potato
and cut into chips. Scatter on a baking tray
and cover in coconut oil and spices. Bake for
20 minutes, or until the chips are crispy.

5   Heat the coconut oil in a large frying pan
and fry the patties for 2–3 minutes each side,
then place on a baking tray in the oven for
10–15 minutes, or until cooked through.

6   To serve, place the spinach, tomato, avocado and
feta inside two big lettuce leaves and top with a
patty. Serve with sweet potato chips and sauce
of your preference. We love mustard!

MAKES 8 PATTIES

Vegan option

REPLACE THE CHICKEN
BURGERS WITH ROAST
VEGGIE PATTIES
(SEE RECIPE PAGE 170).

188 Totally Buf

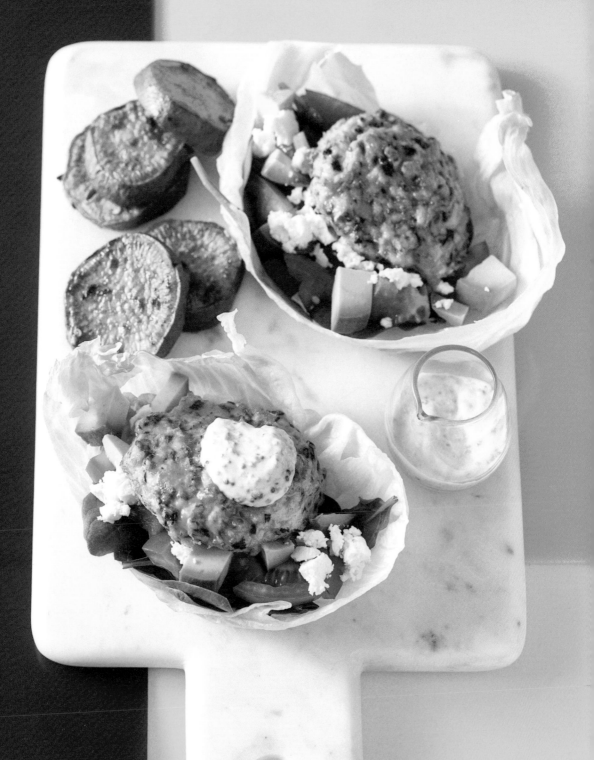

Chicken-stuffed Sweet Potatoes

Beautiful

2 medium sweet potatoes,
   scrubbed
½ leek, washed and thinly sliced
2 cups tightly packed spinach
   leaves
1 cup finely chopped broccoli
½ cup shredded Brussels sprouts,
   trimmed and outer leaves
   discarded

Unstoppable

300 g chicken breast, diced

Fearless

½ tablespoon coconut oil
1 teaspoon sea salt
¼ teaspoon pepper
feta and olives, to serve (optional)

1   Preheat the oven to 160°C and line a tray with
    baking paper.

2   Rub the skins of the sweet potatoes all over
    with the coconut oil and sprinkle them with salt.
    Prick with a fork a few times and place on the
    baking tray. Bake until tender, about 40 minutes.

3   Place a large frying pan over medium-high
    heat and sauté the leek for 5 minutes. Add the
    remaining ingredients (except the cooked sweet
    potato) and continue sautéing until the chicken
    is cooked through and the vegetables are
    softened, about 10 minutes.

4   Scoop a little flesh out of the sweet potatoes
    and fill them with the chicken mixture.

5   Serve with feta and olives, if you like.

SERVES 2

Vegan option

SAUTÉ THE VEGETABLES
WITH RED KIDNEY BEANS
INSTEAD OF CHICKEN, AND
FILL THE SWEET POTATOES
WITH THE MIX.

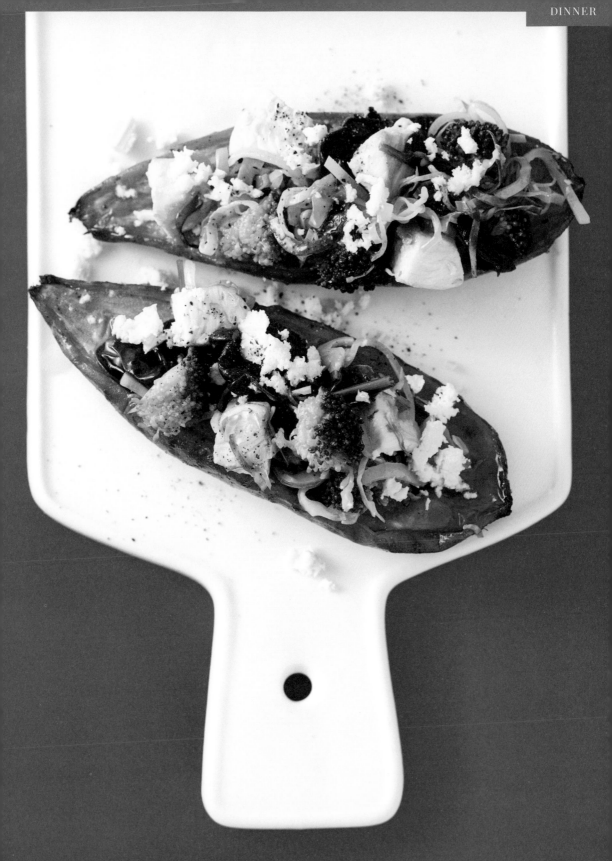

Cumin-spiced Meatballs with Carrot 'Pasta'

Beautiful

4 carrots, spiralised (for 'pasta')

½ cup roughly chopped parsley

Unstoppable

500 g beef mince

1 egg

1 tablespoon sesame seeds

Fearless

1 tablespoon ground cumin

1 teaspoon curry powder

½ teaspoon sea salt

1 tablespoon olive oil

AVOCADO SAUCE

1 ripe avocado

¼ cup coconut cream

juice of ½ lemon

½ cup roughly chopped coriander

¼ cup water

1 chilli

1 teaspoon salt

1 In a bowl, mix together the beef mince, egg, cumin, curry powder and salt. Roll into small balls.

2 Heat the oil in a frying pan and cook the meatballs for 10 minutes, or until fully cooked.

3 To make the avocado sauce, simply place all the sauce ingredients in a blender and whiz until well combined.

4 Serve the meatballs over the carrot 'pasta', top with avocado sauce and sprinkle with the parsley.

SERVES 4

Vegan option

USE OUR VEGGIE PATTY MIX (PAGE 170), BUT ROLL IT INTO BALLS INSTEAD!

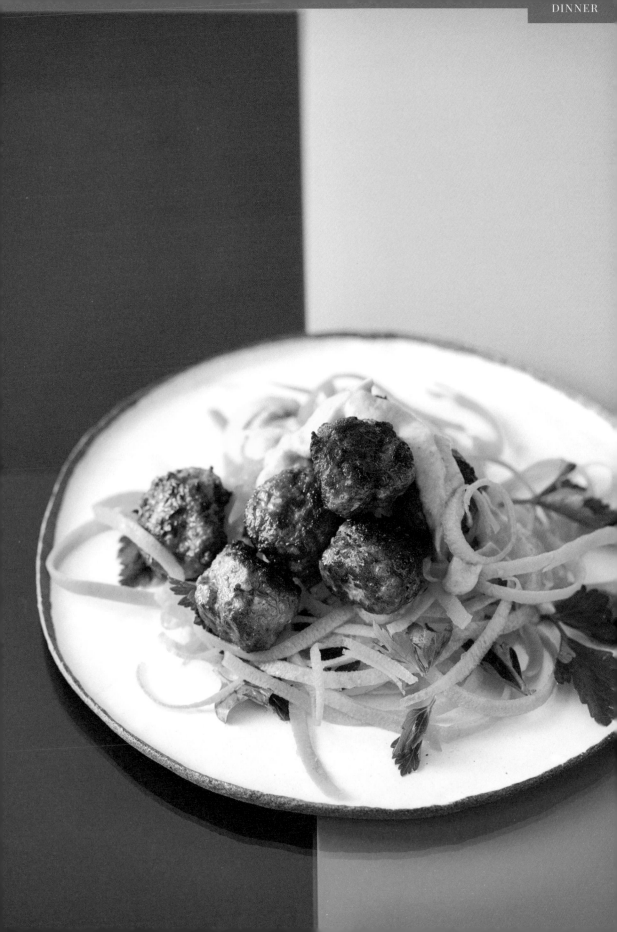

Hearty Bolognese with Zucchini 'Pasta'

Beautiful

½ leek, washed and thinly sliced

1 carrot, grated

1 tomato, diced

1 handful of green beans, trimmed
   and sliced

100 g mushrooms, sliced

3 cloves garlic, crushed

1 handful of Italian parsley

1½ zucchini, spiralised (for 'pasta')

Unstoppable

250–300 g beef mince

sprinkle of Parmesan (optional)

Fearless

2 tablespoons coconut oil

2 tablespoons dulse flakes

1 tablespoon ground cumin

1 tablespoon ground turmeric

400 g can crushed tomatoes

2 tablespoons tomato paste

1 tablespoon vegetable or chicken
   stock powder

sea salt and pepper, to taste

1　Place a large frying pan over medium-high heat and melt the coconut oil. Add the leek and sauté for 3–4 minutes, then add the beef mince, breaking it up in the pan using a wooden spoon. Cook for a further 8–10 minutes.

2　Add the dulse flakes, carrot, tomato, beans and mushrooms and cook for 4 minutes, or until the vegetables have softened. Add the garlic, cumin, turmeric, tinned tomatoes, tomato paste, stock and parsley and season with salt and pepper. If the sauce is very thick, add a little boiling water.

3　Bring the sauce to the boil then simmer for 10 minutes with the lid on. Let it stand for 30 minutes before serving, allowing the sauce to thicken and the flavours to intensify.

4　To serve, divide the spiralised zucchini between two bowls and top with the Bolognese and, if you like, a little Parmesan.

SERVES 2

Vegan option

INSTEAD OF BEEF MINCE,
USE LENTILS, RED BEANS
OR SILKEN TOFU.

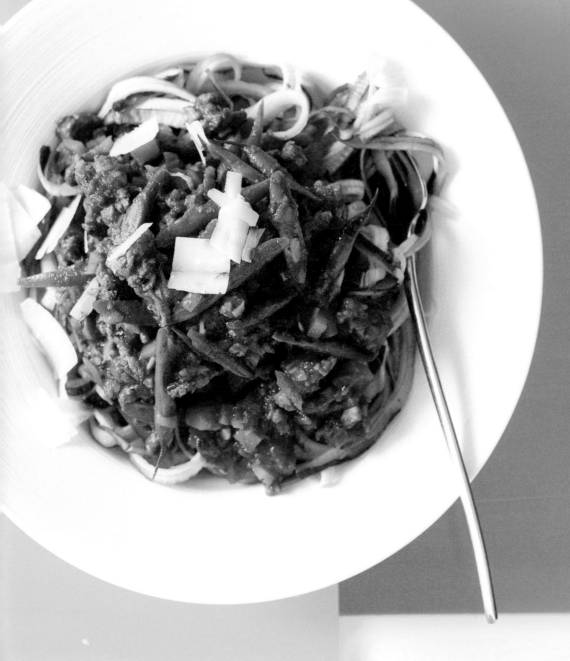

♥ Buf Girls' fave!

Kale and Mushroom Rice with Chicken

Beautiful

1 red onion, diced
2 cloves garlic, crushed
200 g button mushrooms,
    quartered
2 cups roughly chopped kale
1 cup diced broccoli
¼ cup roughly chopped parsley
¼ cup roughly chopped dill

Unstoppable

½ cup brown rice (yields 1½ cups
    cooked rice)
250 g chicken breast, cut into
    cubes

Fearless

1 tablespoon olive oil
2 cups vegetable stock
sea salt and pepper, to taste

1 Cook the rice first. Place the rice in a saucepan
   with 1½ cups of water and simmer for 30 minutes.
   You may need to add a dash more water in the
   cooking process.

2 Place a large frying pan over medium heat,
   add the olive oil and cook the onion and garlic
   for 3 minutes, or until the onion becomes
   translucent. Next, add the chicken and cook
   for 5 minutes. Add the mushrooms, kale and
   broccoli and cook for a further 5 minutes, until
   the mushrooms are softened. Finally, add the
   vegetable stock and rice and cook for
   10 minutes.

3 Stir in the parsley and dill, season with salt
   and pepper, and serve.

SERVES 4

Vegan option

REPLACE THE CHICKEN
WITH TEMPEH, OR ADD
SOME KIDNEY BEANS.

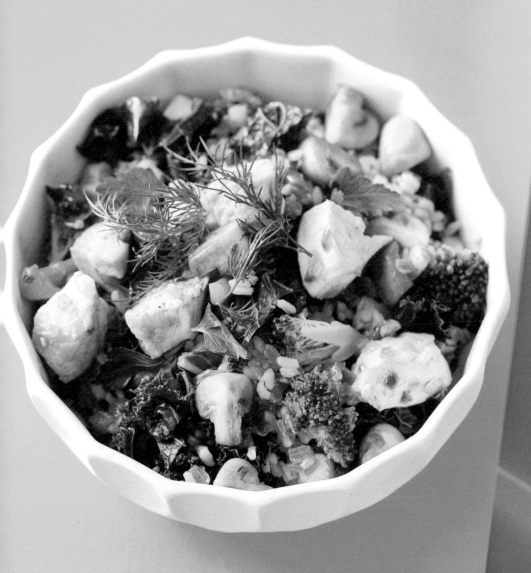

Mexican Mince and Bean Bowl

Beautiful

1 carrot, grated
1 small red chilli, finely chopped
1 head of cos lettuce, roughly
   chopped
8 cherry tomatoes, halved
1 red capsicum, finely chopped
¼ red onion, finely diced
½ cup roughly chopped coriander
½ lemon

Unstoppable

250 g beef mince
200 g (½ can) black beans, drained
   and rinsed
toasted flatbread (optional)

Fearless

1 teaspoon smoked paprika
1 tablespoon olive oil
½ avocado, mashed
sea salt and pepper, to taste

1 Place a frying pan over high heat, add the olive oil and fry the beef mince for 5 minutes, or until it starts to brown. Add the carrot, chilli and paprika and continue cooking until the mince is fully cooked. Season with salt and pepper.

2 Layer the lettuce, tomato, capsicum, red onion and black beans in a serving bowl, spoon the mince on top and scatter with avocado, coriander and a squeeze of lemon juice. Serve with a side of toasted flatbread, if desired.

SERVES 2

Vegan option

REPLACE THE MINCE
WITH BROWN RICE.

Pair this with our
Mock Mojito
[PAGE 244]
for a **Mexican**
feast!

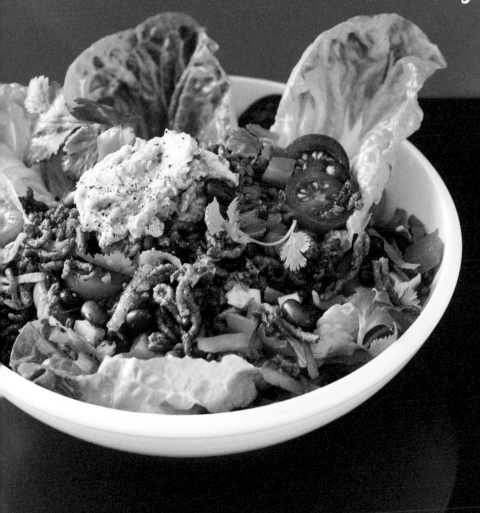

Mexican Stuffed Capsicums

Beautiful

1 onion, diced
2 cloves garlic, minced
1 celery stick, diced
1 carrot, diced
2 kale leaves, stalks removed and
 leaves shredded
1 zucchini, diced
½ punnet cherry tomatoes, halved
4 large red capsicums

Unstoppable

500 g beef mince
400 g can kidney beans, drained
 and rinsed

Fearless

1 tablespoon olive oil
3 teaspoons ground cumin
2 teaspoons ground turmeric
1 teaspoon paprika
2 tablespoons tomato paste
2 tablespoons chopped jalapeños
sea salt and pepper, to taste
lime wedges, to serve
1 handful of coriander leaves, to
 serve
finely sliced chilli, to serve
sprinkle of sheep's or goat's feta,
 to serve

1 Heat a large frying pan over medium heat and drizzle with the olive oil. Add the onion and garlic and sauté for 2 minutes. Add the celery and carrot and sauté for a further 3 minutes.

2 Add the beef mince to the pan and break it up using a wooden spoon. Sprinkle over the cumin, turmeric and paprika and stir well. Once the mince is browned, add the kale, zucchini, tomato, kidney beans, tomato paste and jalapeños, and season with salt and pepper.

3 Reduce the heat and simmer for 15–20 minutes.

4 Preheat the oven to 160°C.

5 Slice the top from each capsicum and remove all seeds and white membrane. Arrange the capsicums on a baking tray. Spoon the mince filling into each and bake for 15 minutes, or until the capsicum is tender.

6 Serve with lime, coriander, chilli and feta.

SERVES 2

Vegan option

SIMPLY LEAVE OUT THE MINCE,
OR SWAP FOR DICED MUSHROOM –
IT'S STILL TOTALLY DELICIOUS!

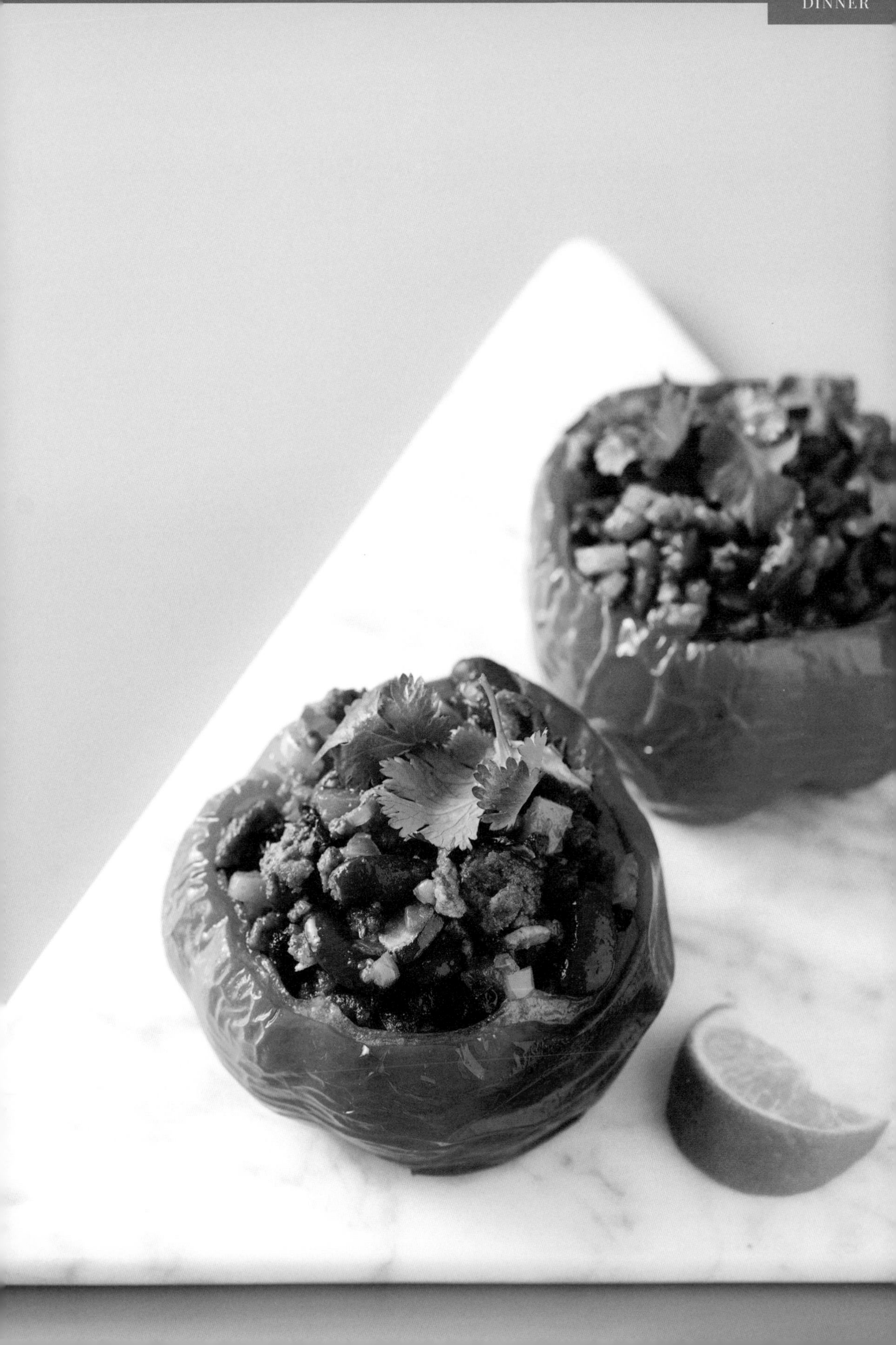

Mushroom and Cauliflower Pizza

Beautiful

¼ cauliflower, whizzed in a food
    processor to make cauliflower
    'rice'
1 handful of mushrooms, sliced
½ leek, washed, sliced and diced
1 handful of rocket

Unstoppable

1–2 eggs plus 1–2 egg whites
    (you can also just use 2 whole
    eggs or vegan egg substitute)
⅓ cup shaved Parmesan
    (or nutritional yeast flakes)

Fearless

1 tablespoon coconut oil
1 teaspoon ground turmeric
sea salt and pepper, to taste
1 tablespoon butter or olive oil

1   Preheat the oven to 180°C.

2   Place an ovenproof frying pan over high heat,
    add the coconut oil, cauliflower, turmeric and
    a little salt, and sauté until the cauliflower
    is cooked through but not yet caramelised.
    Remove from the pan and allow to cool.

3   In the same hot pan, sauté the mushroom and
    leek in the butter until caramelised. Season with
    salt and pepper. Remove from the pan.

4   Mix the eggs and cauliflower together in a bowl
    until well combined. Return the frying pan to
    low-medium heat and pour in the egg and
    cauliflower mixture, allowing it to spread across
    the pan. Cook until almost cooked through and
    slightly browned on the bottom.

5   Sprinkle the mushroom and leek mixture over
    the egg 'pizza base' and scatter most of the
    Parmesan on top. Place under a grill for several
    minutes, until the cheese has melted.

6   Remove from the grill, top with rocket and the
    remaining Parmesan.

MAKES 1 PIZZA

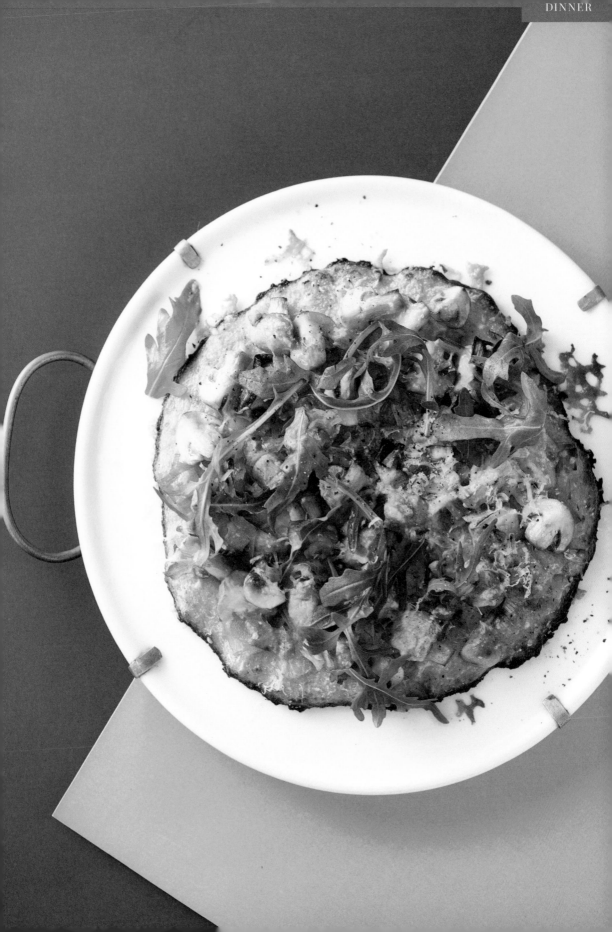

Mushroom and Chicken Pesto Stacks

Beautiful

2 large portobello mushrooms,
stalks removed
1 red capsicum, deseeded and
thinly sliced
juice and zest of 1 lemon
2 cups rocket

Unstoppable

1 chicken breast, sliced in half

Fearless

2 tablespoons olive oil
1 tablespoon mixed herbs
2 tablespoons pesto (store-bought
or Rocket Pesto – see recipe
page 243)
sea salt and pepper, to taste

1   In a large bowl, place the chicken breast,
mushrooms, capsicum, lemon juice, lemon
zest, olive oil, mixed herbs, salt and pepper.
Use your hands to combine, and marinate in the
refrigerator for 30 minutes.

2   Preheat the oven to 180°C and line a tray with
baking paper. Tip the contents of the bowl onto
the tray and bake for 20 minutes, or until the
chicken is cooked through.

3   To serve the stacks, place a mushroom on each
plate and top with pesto, rocket, chicken and
finally capsicum.

SERVES 2

Vegan option

REPLACE THE CHICKEN
WITH SLICES OF TOASTED
SWEET POTATO – LITERALLY
JUST SLICE YOUR SWEET
POTATO AND PUT IN YOUR
TOASTER FOR 2–3 CYCLES
UNTIL COOKED THROUGH.

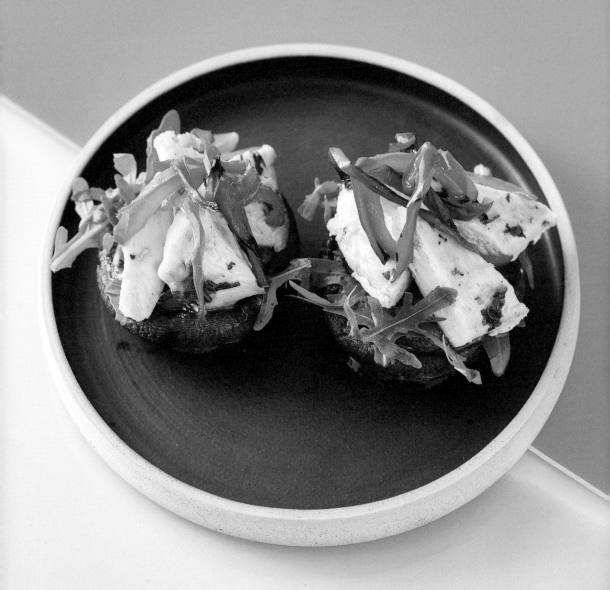

Oven-baked Fish and Chips

Beautiful

1 large beetroot

1 small sweet potato

1 carrot

2 tablespoons roughly chopped
   dill, or herbs of your choice

1 lemon, sliced

2 cups of salad leaves
   (e.g. spinach or rocket), to serve

Unstoppable

2 x white fish fillets
   (about 150 g each)

Fearless

2 tablespoons olive oil

1 teaspoon paprika

sea salt and pepper, to taste

1   Wash the beetroot, sweet potato and carrot well, then cut into thin chips.

2   Preheat the oven to 180°C and line a large tray with baking paper.

3   In a bowl, toss together the cut vegetables with 1 tablespoon of the olive oil, plus the paprika, salt and pepper. Tip onto the baking tray and bake for 15 minutes.

4   While the vegetables are cooking, cut two large squares of aluminium foil and place a fish fillet on each. Drizzle with the remaining olive oil, garnish with chopped dill and arrange the lemon slices on top. Fold the aluminium foil over to form parcels for the fish.

5   At the 15-minute mark, remove the vegetables from the oven, make room in the centre of the baking tray and transfer the fish parcels to the tray. Return the tray to the oven and bake for another 15 minutes, or until the fish is cooked through.

6   Serve with the side of salad leaves.

SERVES 2

Vegan option

SWAP THE FISH FOR
A TOFU STEAK

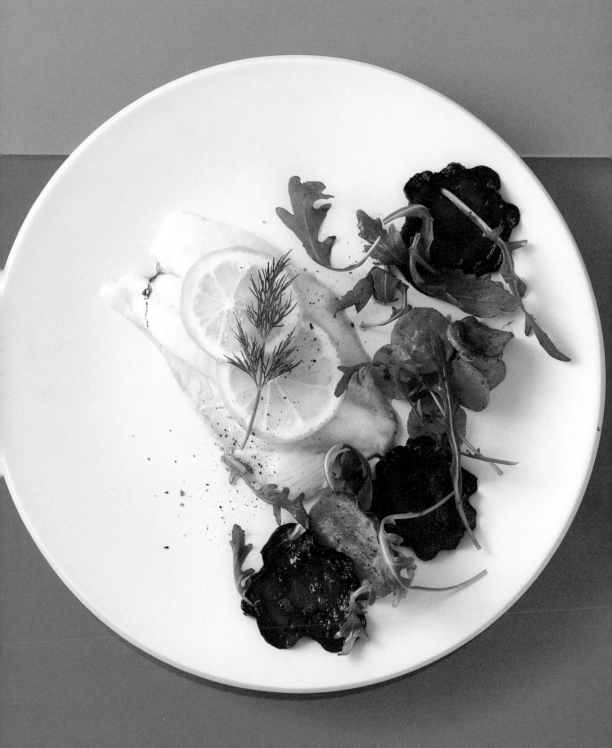

Pan-fried Salmon with Sautéed Greens

Beautiful

1 bunch broccolini, trimmed and
cut in half
1 cup green beans, topped and
tailed
1 cup roughly chopped kale
1 lemon

Unstoppable

2 x salmon fillets (about 150 g
each)
¼ cup dukkah, to season

Fearless

1 tablespoon olive oil
sea salt and pepper, to taste

1 To cook the salmon, place a frying pan over
high heat, add the olive oil and cook the salmon
for 5 minutes each side, or until cooked to your
liking. TIP: rub salt into the skin of the salmon
10 minutes before cooking to make it extra
crispy! Once cooked, remove from the pan and
place on paper towels to drain any excess oil.

2 In the same pan, sauté the broccolini, beans and
kale, adding a dash of water to help them cook.
Cook for 3–4 minutes or until the vegetables are
tender.

3 Top the vegetables with dukkah and serve
alongside the salmon. To finish, squeeze over
the lemon and season with salt and pepper.

SERVES 2

Vegan option

DITCH THE SALMON AND
REPLACE WITH A BIG WEDGE
OF CINNAMON ROASTED
PUMPKIN (SEE RECIPE PAGE
242), OR BROWN RICE AND
A DRIZZLE OF TAHINI.

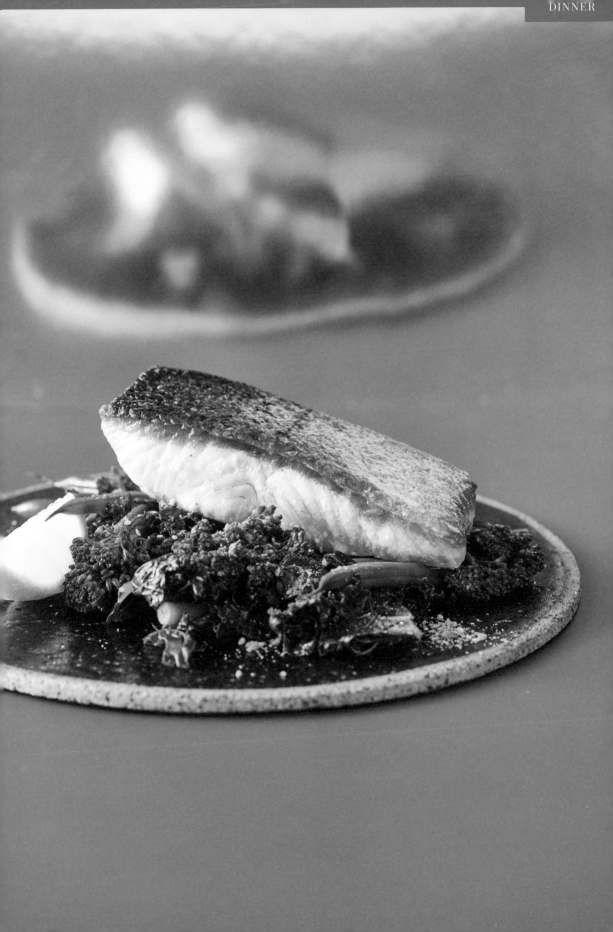

Pan-fried Steak with Sautéed Greens

Beautiful

1 bunch broccolini, trimmed
   and cut in half
1 cup snow peas, trimmed
2 cups spinach leaves
1 lemon

Unstoppable

2 x grass-fed steaks
   (about 150 g each)

Fearless

1 tablespoon olive oil
sea salt and pepper, to taste

1   Place a frying pan over high heat, add the olive oil and cook the steaks for 3–5 minutes each side, or until cooked to your liking. Once cooked, remove from the pan, squeeze over half the lemon juice and cover with foil while you prepare the greens.

2   In the same pan, sauté the broccolini, snow peas and spinach with a dash of water and the remaining lemon juice. Cook for 3–4 minutes, until vegetables are tender.

3   Slice the steak into thin strips, season with salt and pepper and serve with the greens.

SERVES 2

Vegan option

REPLACE THE STEAK WITH 2 CHUNKY PIECES OF RYE SOURDOUGH SPREAD WITH ALMOND BUTTER. IT'S SO DELICIOUS WITH THE GREENS!

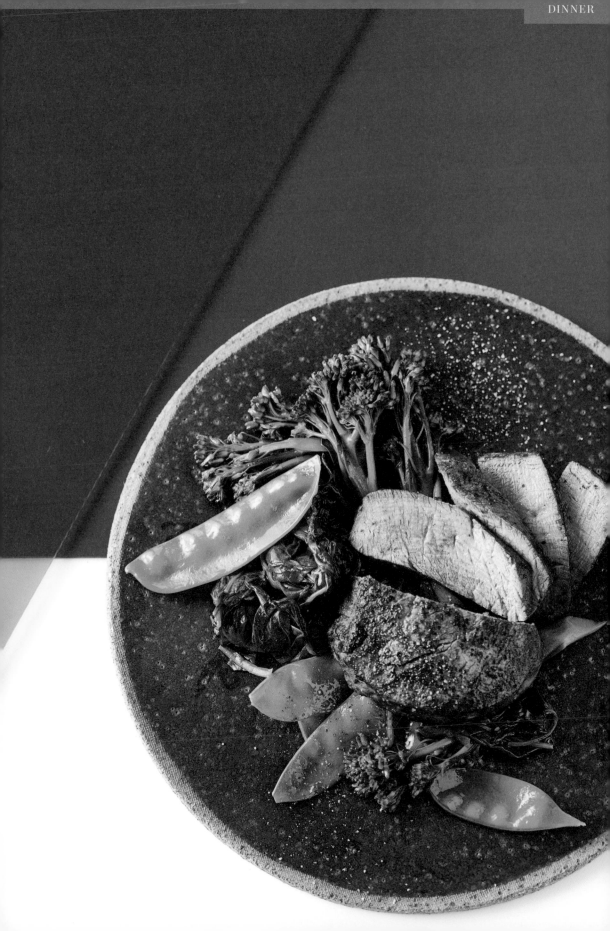

Raw Pad Thai

Beautiful

1 carrot, spiralised

1 zucchini, spiralised

1 cup finely chopped purple cabbage

1 red capsicum, thinly sliced

100 g snow peas, topped and tailed and thinly sliced

½ cup roughly chopped coriander

1 lime, to serve

Unstoppable

¼ cup roughly chopped roasted almonds

Fearless

SATAY SAUCE

1 tablespoon lemon juice

1 teaspoon grated fresh ginger

1 tablespoon honey or maple syrup

¼ cup almond butter

1 tablespoon tahini

2 tablespoons tamari

1 In a large bowl, combine the carrot, zucchini, cabbage, capsicum, snow peas and coriander.

2 In a separate bowl, mix together all the Satay Sauce ingredients. The sauce will be quite thick.

3 Pour the sauce onto the salad and, using your hands, toss until the salad is dressed well.

4 Dish up the salad into two bowls and top with the almonds and a squeeze of lime juice.

SERVES 2

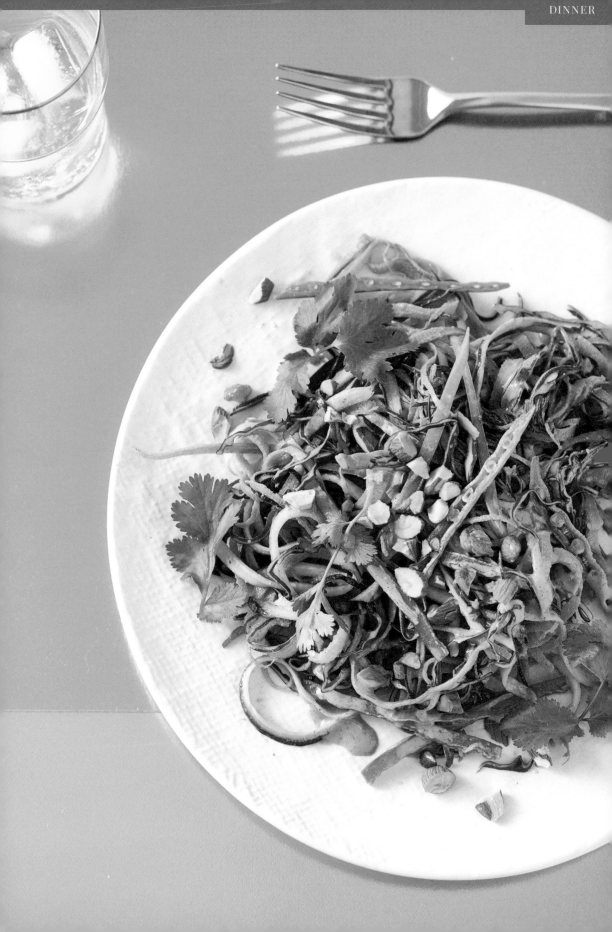

Ricotta and Mushroom Zucchetti

Beautiful

2 cloves garlic, crushed

1 red onion, finely diced

200 g button mushrooms,
   quartered

2 cups finely chopped silverbeet

½ cup spinach leaves

½ cup roughly chopped basil

4 zucchini, spiralised

juice of ½ lemon

Unstoppable

¾ cup ricotta

¼ cup almond or coconut milk

Fearless

1 tablespoon olive oil

sea salt and pepper, to taste

1   Heat the oil in a large frying pan over medium heat. Add the garlic, onion and mushrooms and cook for 5 minutes, or until the onion becomes translucent.

2   In a bowl, mix together the ricotta, almond milk, salt and pepper. Pour into the frying pan and allow the mixture to come to a simmer. Continue cooking for 4–5 minutes.

3   Add the silverbeet, spinach and basil and cook until the silverbeet is wilted. Season with extra salt and pepper, if required, and the lemon juice.

4   Toss through the spiralised zucchini for 3 minutes, until warmed, and serve into bowls.

SERVES 4

Vegan option

LEAVE OUT THE RICOTTA, BUT BE AWARE THAT THE MIXTURE WON'T BE AS THICK AS THE ORIGINAL RECIPE, SO YOU MAY WANT TO ADD A SUBSTITUTE, LIKE A GENEROUS DASH OF COCONUT CREAM.

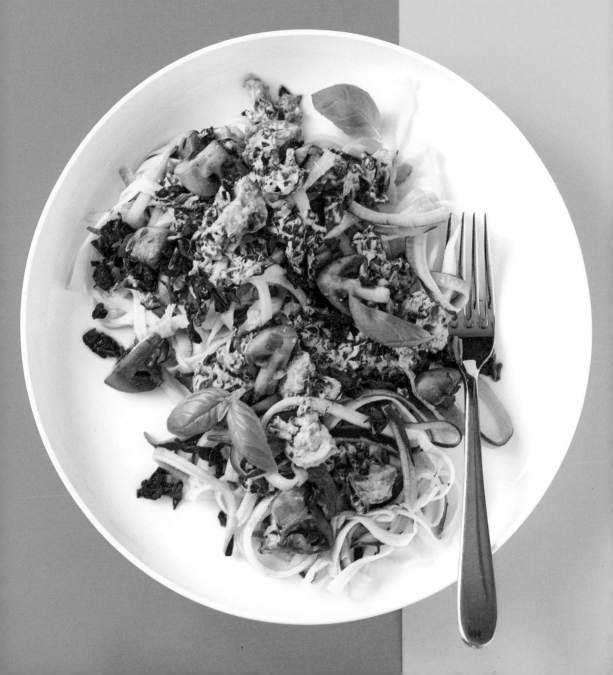

Roast Chicken with Carrot and Pumpkin Purée

Beautiful

600 g pumpkin, cut into 2 cm cubes
(keep the skin on for extra fibre)
2 carrots, roughly chopped
3 cloves garlic, skins removed
zest and juice of 1 lemon

Unstoppable

1 whole chicken

Fearless

2 tablespoons olive oil
1 sprig of rosemary, chopped
1 teaspoon smoked paprika
sea salt and pepper, to taste
½ cup coconut cream

1   Preheat the oven to 180°C and line two trays with baking paper.

2   Prepare the chicken for roasting by rubbing 1 tablespoon of oil, and salt and pepper, into the skin. Coat with the lemon juice and zest and sprinkle with rosemary. Place chicken in the oven to roast for 1 hour, or until juices run clear.

3   Meanwhile, place the pumpkin and carrot in the second baking tray and toss with the garlic cloves, the remaining oil, and salt and pepper. Roast for 25 minutes, or until the vegetables are golden and soft.

4   Allow the veggies to cool slightly then whiz in a blender with the coconut cream and paprika to make a purée. Season with extra salt and pepper, if desired.

5   Once the chicken is cooked, remove from the oven and carve into portions. Serve on a bed of purée and drizzle with the lemon juice.

SERVES 4

Vegan option

PREPARE 4 TOFU STEAKS FOLLOWING STEP 2, BUT BAKE FOR 30 MINUTES.

Buf Girls' Tip

DON'T FEEL LIKE CHICKEN? YOU CAN SIMPLY MAKE THE ROAST CARROT AND PUMPKIN PURÉE ON ITS OWN AND HAVE IT AS A DIP. USE LESS COCONUT CREAM FOR A THICKER CONSISTENCY.

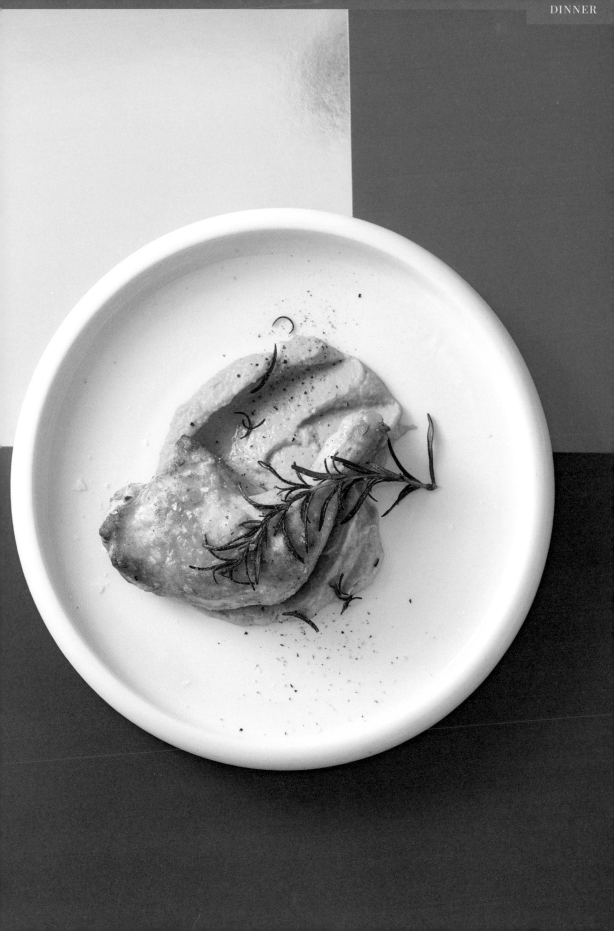

San Choy Bao Balls

Beautiful

1 carrot, grated
1 tablespoon grated fresh ginger
1 teaspoon chilli flakes
2 tablespoons thinly sliced spring
   onion
¼ cup roughly chopped coriander
1 lime
leaves of 1 iceberg lettuce, to serve
1 cup alfalfa, to serve

Unstoppable

500 g chicken mince
1 egg

Fearless

1 tablespoon tamari
1 tablespoon coconut oil

DIPPING SAUCE
2 tablespoons tahini
1 tablespoon tamari
½ tablespoon honey
juice of ½ lime
1 tablespoon water

1 In a bowl, combine the carrot, ginger, chilli flakes, spring onion, coriander, chicken mince, egg, tamari and the juice of half the lime. Mix well and then roll mixture into 16 balls.

2 Heat a frying pan over medium heat, add the coconut oil and fry the balls, turning regularly until fully cooked through, for about 8–10 minutes.

3 To make the dressing, simply mix all the Dipping Sauce ingredients together.

4 Choose eight iceberg lettuce leaves that resemble cups and fill each with a portion of alfalfa, and two san choy bao balls.

5 To serve, squeeze over the juice of the remaining lime half and drizzle with a spoonful of the dipping sauce.

SERVES 4

Vegan option

REPLACE THE CHICKEN BALLS WITH OUR TRIPLE C VEGGIE PATTIES (PAGE 174).

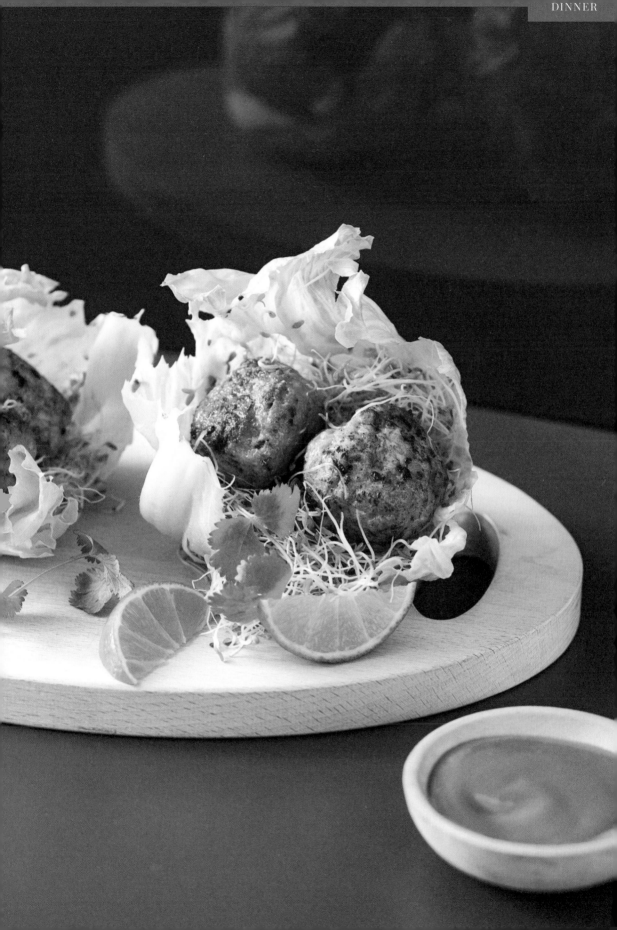

Sweet Potato Chicken Curry

Beautiful

1 onion, diced
2 cloves garlic, crushed
1 tablespoon grated fresh ginger
1 sweet potato, cut into small
    cubes
1 zucchini, diced
½ cup roughly chopped coriander,
    to serve

Unstoppable

400 g chicken breast, diced

Fearless

1 tablespoon olive oil
1 tablespoon curry powder
400 ml coconut milk
sea salt and pepper, to taste

1. Place a large frying pan over medium-high heat, add the olive oil and sauté the onion and garlic for 3–4 minutes, or until the onion becomes translucent. Add the chicken and cook for 5 minutes, or until browned. Add the ginger and curry powder and cook for 2 minutes, until fragrant. Add the coconut milk, sweet potato and zucchini and bring to a simmer.

2. Cover with a lid and simmer for 15–20 minutes, or until the sweet potatoes are tender. Season with salt and pepper and serve with coriander sprinkled on top.

SERVES 4

Vegan option

REPLACE THE CHICKEN
WITH ½ CUP EACH OF
KIDNEY BEANS AND
BROWN RICE.

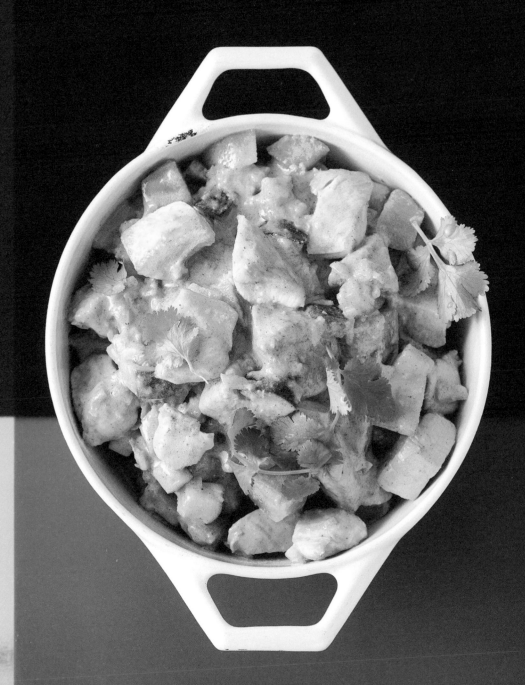

Sweet Potato Gnocchi

Beautiful

800 g sweet potato (about 3–4 medium-sized sweet potatoes)

Unstoppable

1 egg yolk (or vegan egg substitute)

¼ cup freshly grated Parmesan (or nutritional yeast flakes) (optional)

2 cups gluten-free flour (e.g. brown rice flour or coconut flour)

Fearless

cracked black pepper, to serve

1 Peel the sweet potato, chop into chunks and cook until soft. You can choose how you want to cook it: roasting and steaming both work well. Once cooked, mash the sweet potato until smooth. Transfer to a large mixing bowl and leave to cool for 15–20 minutes.

2 Combine the cooled sweet potato mash with the egg yolk and Parmesan, then gradually sift in the flour until you get a non-sticky dough mixture. (You might find that you use less than 2 cups, which is totally fine!)

3 Dust your kitchen bench with a little flour and transfer the dough to the bench. Knead for a few minutes, then divide the mixture into four equal portions and roll each portion into a sausage shape (you want it to be around 3 cm thick). Slice each sausage into 3 cm pieces.

4 To cook your gnocchi, add to a pan of boiling water. When it floats to the top, it's ready! Top with your favourite sauce, and vegetables on the side, season with black pepper and serve.

SERVES 4

Buf Girls' Tip

SAUCE IDEAS INCLUDE FRESH PESTO (SEE RECIPE PAGE 247), HEARTY BOLOGNESE WITH ZUCCHINI PASTA (MINUS THE SPIRALISED ZUCCHINI — SEE RECIPE PAGE 194) AND ARRABBIATA SAUCE.

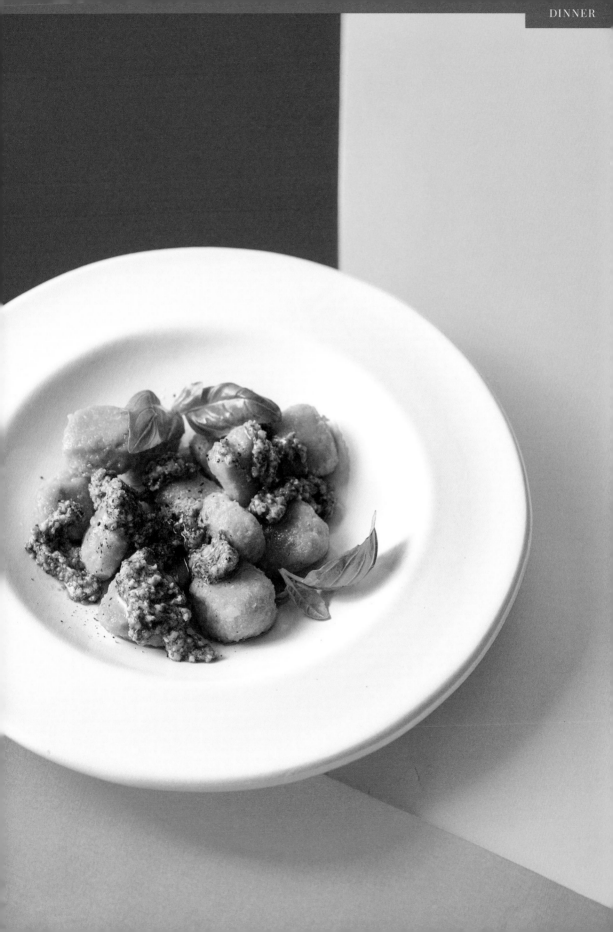

The 'Orange' Soup

Beautiful

800 g pumpkin, cut into cubes
4 large carrots, cut into cubes
2 cloves garlic, crushed
1 onion, roughly chopped

Unstoppable

½ cup raw, unsalted peanuts

Fearless

2 tablespoons olive oil
1 tablespoon curry powder
sea salt and pepper, to taste
400 ml coconut milk
1 litre vegetable stock

1 Preheat the oven to 180°C and line a tray with baking paper.

2 In a large bowl, toss the pumpkin, carrots, garlic, onion, olive oil, curry powder and salt and pepper together until well coated.

3 Spread the vegetables onto the baking tray and bake for 20 minutes. Remove from the oven, sprinkle the peanuts on top and bake for another 10 minutes, until the peanuts are roasted.

4 Return the baked vegetables to the bowl and add the coconut milk and vegetable stock. Transfer batches of the mixture to a blender and whiz until well combined.

SERVES 4–6

Buf Girls' Tip

ADD AN EXTRA SERVE OF (U)NSTOPPABLE PROTEIN SUCH AS PAN-FRIED BACON PIECES OR TOFU.

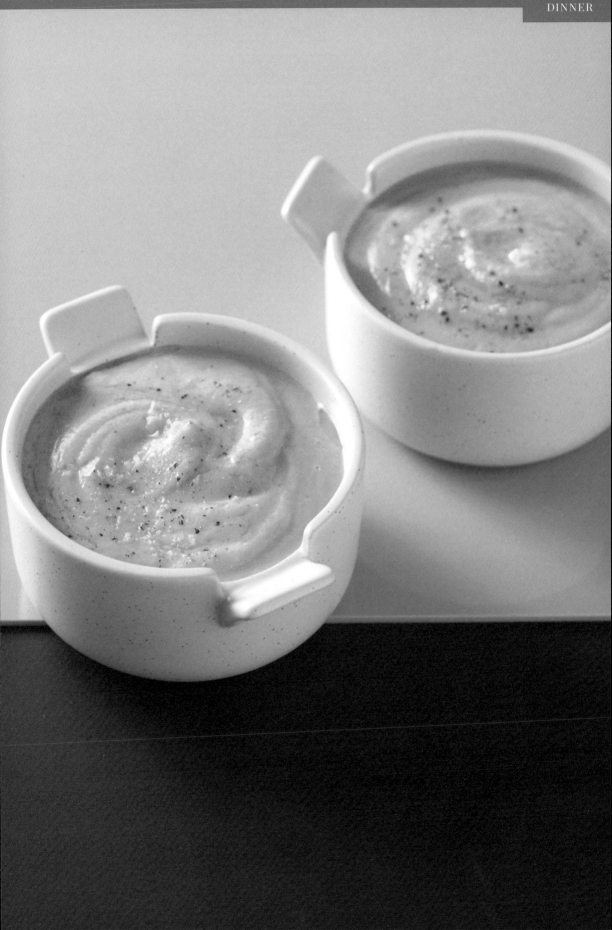

Turmeric, Cauliflower and Egg Salad

Beautiful

½ head of cauliflower, cut into florets

2 cups spinach leaves

juice of ½ lemon

Unstoppable

4 boiled eggs

1 teaspoon honey

Fearless

sea salt and pepper, to taste

½ tablespoon olive oil

½ cup coconut yoghurt

1 teaspoon ground turmeric

1 Steam the cauliflower in a saucepan until tender when pricked with a knife. Allow to cool completely.

2 Peel the boiled eggs and mash them in a bowl.

3 To make a dressing, simply combine the lemon juice, olive oil, yoghurt, turmeric and honey in a bowl.

4 In another bowl, mix together the cauliflower, spinach and eggs. Toss with the dressing and season with salt and pepper.

SERVES 2

Vegan option

REPLACE THE EGGS WITH AVOCADO AND POMEGRANATE SEEDS, OR CHUNKS OF ROASTED PUMPKIN OR SWEET POTATO. SWAP THE HONEY FOR MAPLE SYRUP.

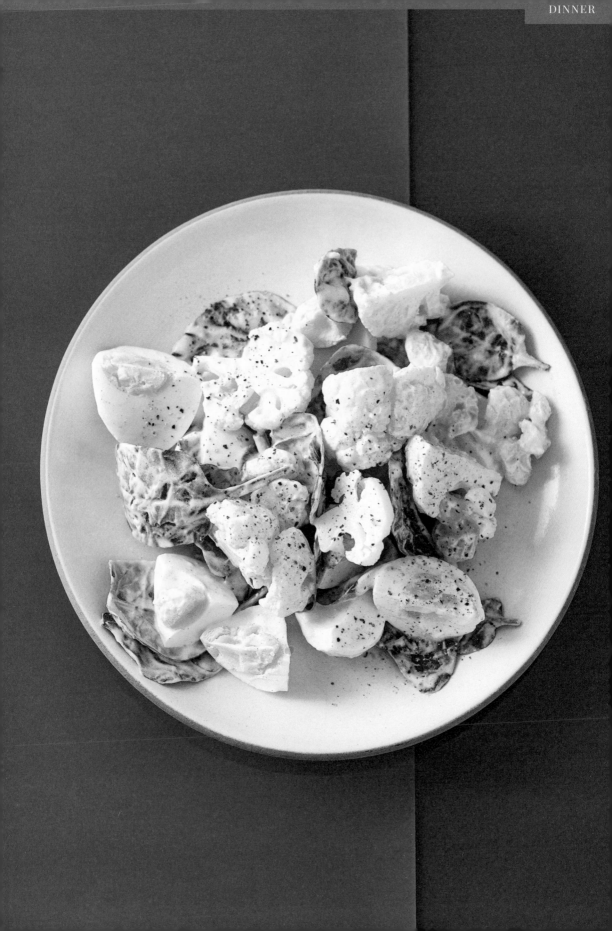

Vegetable Quinoa Curry

Beautiful

1 eggplant, cut into small cubes
1 carrot, diced
1 zucchini, diced
1 onion, diced
2 cloves garlic, crushed

Unstoppable

¾ cup quinoa
½ cup roughly chopped cashews

Fearless

1 tablespoon olive oil
1 tablespoon curry powder
1 teaspoon ground turmeric
1 teaspoon cinnamon
400 g can crushed tomatoes
½ cup coconut cream
sea salt and pepper, to taste

1 Heat the olive oil in a large saucepan and cook the eggplant, carrot, zucchini, onion and garlic for 10-15 minutes, or until the vegetables have softened.

2 Add the curry powder, turmeric and cinnamon and cook for a further 2 minutes. Add the tomato, quinoa and 3 cups of water and bring to the boil. Season with salt and pepper. Once boiling, reduce the heat and simmer for 20 minutes, or until the quinoa is cooked.

3 Before serving, stir through the coconut cream and cashews.

SERVES 4

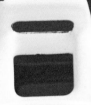
This is
perfect, hearty
soul food!

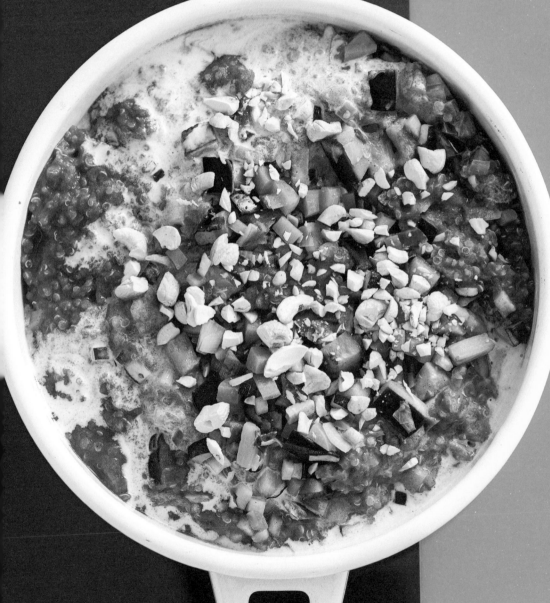

Vegetable Tahini Dream

Beautiful

a mix of non-starchy vegetables
(e.g. broccolini, asparagus, red
capsicum, cherry tomatoes,
zucchini, mushrooms)
a few starchy vegetables (e.g.
sweet potato and beetroot)

Unstoppable

hulled tahini, to taste

Fearless

lemon juice, to taste

1 Chop up all your vegetables, making sure the
   starchy vegetables are in small cubes. The rest
   can be cut chunkily. Steam the vegetables,
   starting with the tubers, which will take about
   15 minutes, then slowly adding in the rest,
   which should take 30–60 seconds. Make sure
   the asparagus goes in last, as it only takes a few
   seconds.

2 Once all vegetables are lightly steamed, pop in
   a bowl, squeeze lemon juice over the top and
   drizzle with a generous amount of tahini.

SERVES AS MANY AS YOU LIKE

Buf Girls' Tip

MAKE A HUGE BATCH
THAT YOU CAN REHEAT AT
ANOTHER MEAL. IT IS IDEAL
ACCOMPANYING SOME LEAN
PROTEIN FOR A LUNCH OR
DINNER, OR JUST TO EAT
AS A SNACK.

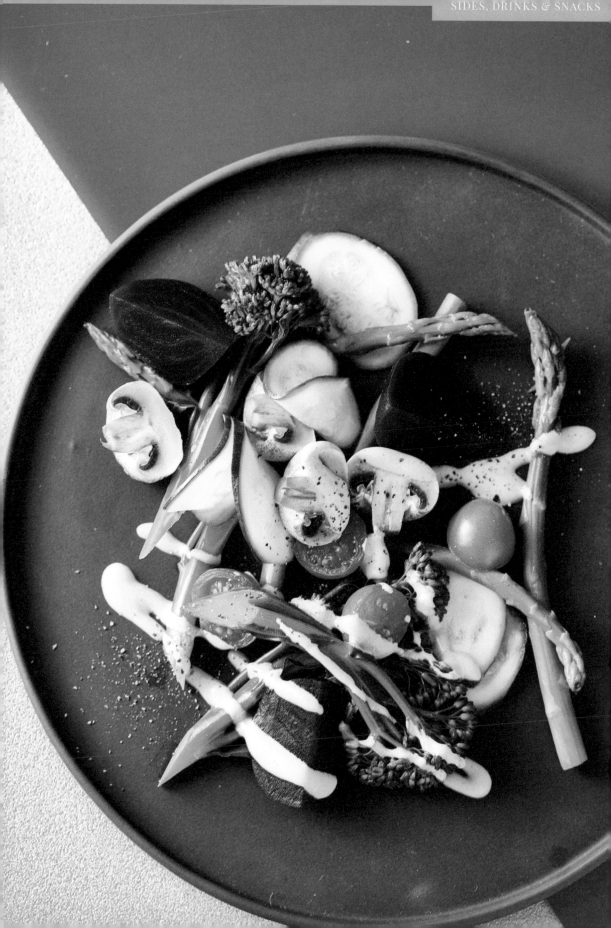

Almond-flour Muffins

Beautiful

1 cup chopped fruits of your choice (see tip)

Unstoppable

1 cup almond meal
2 eggs (or vegan egg substitute)
1 tablespoon maple syrup or honey

Fearless

¼ teaspoon baking soda
½ teaspoon apple cider vinegar
organic butter, to serve

1 Preheat the oven to 180°C.

2 Combine the almond flour and baking soda in a bowl.

3 In a separate bowl, combine the eggs, syrup/honey and vinegar.

4 Stir the dry ingredients into the wet ingredients (plus any extras - see tip below), mixing until combined.

5 Scoop the batter into paper muffin cups and bake for 15 minutes, or until slightly browned around the edges.

6 Allow to cool, then serve with a little butter.

MAKES 4–6

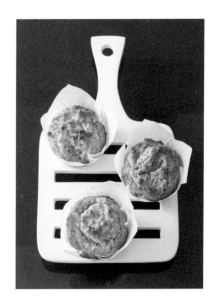

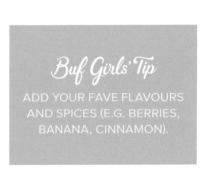

Buf Girls' Tip

ADD YOUR FAVE FLAVOURS AND SPICES (E.G. BERRIES, BANANA, CINNAMON).

Bliss Balls

Beautiful

½ cup chopped pitted dates
(roughly 16) or a big handful
of goji berries

Unstoppable

2 cups mixed nuts of your choice
2 tablespoons honey or
2 tablespoons coconut oil

Fearless

2 tablespoons cacao powder
1 handful of raw cacao nibs
(optional)
desiccated coconut, for sprinkling
and rolling
2–3 tablespoons water

1 Place the nuts, dates, cacao powder and cacao nibs, as well as a sprinkle of the coconut, into a large mixing bowl. Drizzle the honey on top and mix until well combined (this is best done with your hands and will take a bit of effort!), adding water slowly until the mixture becomes a little sticky.

2 Pour the remaining desiccated coconut onto a plate.

3 Take a small amount of the choc mix and roll it into a ball. Now roll it in the coconut until covered. Continue until the entire mix has been used up, then place your balls in the fridge to set.

MAKES 10–12 BALLS

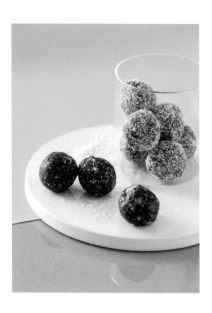

Chocolate Mousse

Beautiful
2 soft avocados

Unstoppable
1 tablespoon honey or maple syrup

Fearless
¼ cup cacao powder

1. Mash the flesh of the avocados and put in a bowl. Add the honey and cacao.
2. Whisk by hand, or purée with an electric mixer, until super-smooth. Refrigerate for a minimum of 3 hours.

Buf Girls' Tip
TOP WITH STRAWBERRIES AND YOGHURT AND LAYER CRUSHED NUTS AT THE BOTTOM OF THE MOUSSE FOR A DELICIOUS SURPRISE WHEN EATING.

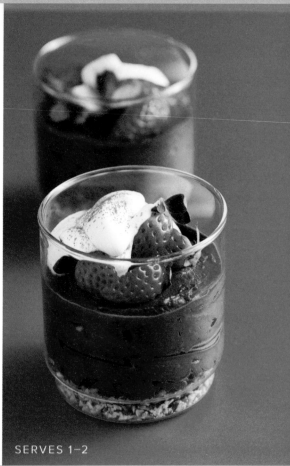

SERVES 1–2

SERVES 1

Buf Girls' Tip
IF YOU NEED TO SWEETEN THIS UP, A DASH OF MAPLE SYRUP OR A LITTLE STEVIA POWDER WORKS WONDERS.

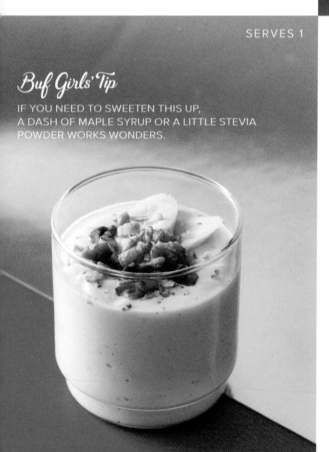

Pro Yoghurt

Beautiful
½ cup frozen mixed berries, or a banana, sliced

Unstoppable
½–1 cup natural yoghurt or coconut yoghurt
1 serve of protein powder
¼ cup nuts/seeds of your choice

Fearless
½–1 tablespoon cacao powder, or cinnamon and a scraped vanilla bean
1 tablespoon shredded coconut (optional)

1. Scoop some yoghurt into a small bowl. Add the protein powder and mix well. If you're a choc-lover, stir in some raw cacao. Vanilla-holics can add a few pinches of cinnamon and some vanilla.
2. Top with shredded coconut, berries, sliced banana or any of your faves – nuts or seeds will add an extra protein kick!

Blend 'em Eggs

Beautiful
½ cup chopped broccoli
1 handful of spinach leaves

Unstoppable
2 eggs
1 tablespoon feta (or vegan feta), crumbled

Fearless
1 teaspoon Dijon mustard
sea salt and pepper, to taste
pinch of chilli flakes, to taste

Place the broccoli, spinach, eggs and mustard in a blender and whiz until smooth. Pour mixture into a small baking dish and top with the feta.

Cook in the microwave for 2 minutes on high. Season to taste with salt and pepper and sprinkle over the chilli flakes

Vegan option
REPLACE THE EGGS WITH A VEGAN EGG SUBSTITUTE, OR ½ CUP OF CHICKPEA FLOUR AND ½ CUP OF ALMOND OR COCONUT MILK.

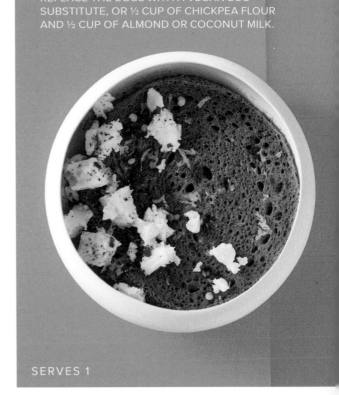

SERVES 1

MAKES AS MANY AS YOU WANT!

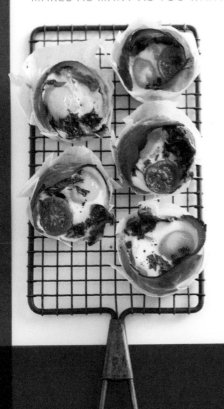

Baked Egg Muffins

Beautiful
spinach leaves, shredded
cherry tomatoes, chopped
mushrooms, sliced

Unstoppable
ham or turkey slices (or soft corn tortillas)
eggs (or a big scoop of hummus)

Fearless
coconut oil spray

1. Preheat the oven to 150°C.
2. Spray a muffin tin with coconut oil. Make a 'muffin case' by criss-crossing slices of ham or turkey or corn tortilla in each muffin hole.
3. Add tomato, mushroom and spinach (plus any other vegetables or protein you love). Crack an egg into each muffin hole and bake for 15–20 minutes.

Fudgy Bean Brownies

Beautiful

2 ripe bananas

Unstoppable

400 g can kidney beans, drained
   and rinsed
⅓ cup maple syrup
⅓ cup buckwheat flour
¼ cup chopped almonds

Fearless

¼ cup cacao powder
1 teaspoon cinnamon
¼ cup dark chocolate pieces
   (optional)

1   Preheat the oven to 180°C and line a bread tin
    with baking paper.

2   Place the bananas, kidney beans, maple syrup,
    cacao and cinnamon into a food processor
    and whiz until blended. Add the almonds and
    buckwheat flour and blend again.

3   Pour the batter into the prepared tin, sprinkle
    with dark chocolate, if you like, and bake for
    25–30 minutes, or until a skewer inserted comes
    out clean.

MAKES 8 SLICES

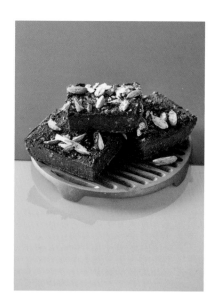

Carob, Banana and Macadamia Loaf

Beautiful

½ cup carob powder

2 ripe bananas, mashed

Unstoppable

¼ cup buckwheat flour

¾ cup almond meal

½ cup roughly chopped
    macadamias

2 eggs, lightly beaten (or vegan
    egg substitute)

¼ cup maple syrup

Fearless

1 teaspoon cinnamon

1 teaspoon baking powder

2 tablespoons coconut oil, melted

1   Preheat the oven to 160°C and line a bread tin
    with baking paper.

2   Place the carob, buckwheat flour, almond meal,
    macadamias, cinnamon and baking powder in a
    large bowl and mix together.

3   In another bowl, combine the banana, eggs,
    maple syrup and coconut oil and mix well.

4   Pour the wet ingredients into the dry ingredients
    and mix until just combined.

5   Pour the mixture into the prepared tin and cook
    in the oven for 35 minutes, or until a skewer
    inserted comes out clean.

MAKES 10 SLICES

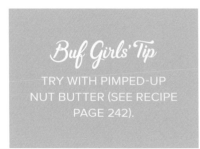

Buf Girls' Tip

TRY WITH PIMPED-UP
NUT BUTTER (SEE RECIPE
PAGE 242).

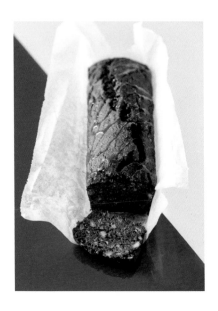

Healthy Strawberry Crumble

Beautiful

500 g hulled strawberries

Unstoppable

40 g almonds
40 g pistachios
5 pitted dates

Fearless

½ teaspoon cinnamon
1 vanilla pod or ½ teaspoon vanilla
   essence

1 Pop your almonds, pistachios, cinnamon and
   three of the dates into a food processor and
   whiz until you have a crumble-like texture. (If
   you don't have a food processor, just finely chop
   the nuts and dates by hand.)

2 For the strawberry mix, if using the vanilla pod,
   slice lengthways and use the knife to scrape the
   seeds. Take 250 g of the strawberries and whiz
   them in the blender along with the vanilla seeds
   (or essence) and the remaining dates. Blend
   until smooth.

3 Cut the remaining strawberries in quarters
   and stir into the blended strawberry mixture.
   Transfer to a dish and top with the crumble mix.

4 If you like it warm, pop the whole thing in the
   oven for 10 minutes at 180°C. The crumble will
   crisp up a bit and be delicious!

SERVES 2–4

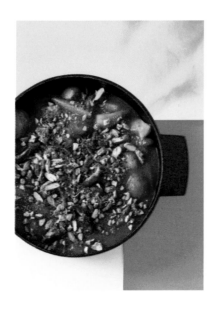

Buf Girls' Tip

THIS RECIPE ALSO WORKS
WELL WITH OTHER FRUITS,
LIKE KIWI, MANGO, MIXED
BERRIES OR A COMBINATION
OF YOUR FAVOURITES.

Oaty Crackers

Beautiful

¼ cup chia seeds
¼ cup sunflower seeds
¼ cup pepitas

Unstoppable

1 cup rolled oats
1 tablespoon maple syrup

Fearless

¼ cup LSA
1 teaspoon sea salt
1 teaspoon mixed dried herbs
1 teaspoon fennel seeds
1 tablespoon coconut oil
¾ cup water

Buf Girls' Tip

SERVE WITH AVOCADO AND CHICKPEA HUMMUS (SEE RECIPE PAGE 243) OR YOUR DIP OF CHOICE. USE THE CRACKERS AS BREAD REPLACEMENTS, OR BREAK THEM UP AND USE AS CROUTONS IN SALADS.

1 Line a large tray with baking paper and cut a second piece of baking paper about the same size.

2 In a bowl, mix together the oats, LSA, chia seeds, sunflower seeds, pepitas, salt, mixed herbs and fennel seeds.

3 In a separate bowl, whisk together the maple syrup, coconut oil and water.

4 Add the wet mixture to the dry mixture and fold through the ingredients. Set aside for 15 minutes to allow the chia seeds and oats to absorb the water and form a pliable mixture.

5 Form the dough into a rough ball and place on the lined tray, flattening slightly with your hands. Place a second piece of baking paper on top and, using a rolling pin, roll out to 3-4 mm thickness. Remove the top sheet of paper and use a butter knife to score squares in the dough. (Don't cut right through the dough - just make an indent.)

6 Preheat the oven to 160°C. Place the tray in the oven for 10 minutes, then remove and carefully flip over the crackers to cook the other side. Return to the oven for another 5-7 minutes, until lightly golden brown. Allow to cool on the tray before removing.

SERVES 6–8

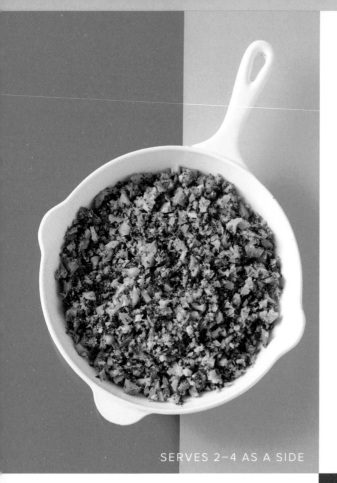

Broccoli Rice

Beautiful
1–2 heads of broccoli
zest of 1 lemon

Unstoppable
1 tablespoon olive or coconut oil

Fearless
sea salt and pepper, to taste

1 Cut the broccoli florets and stalk into small chunks and whiz in a food processor until it resembles small crumbs or 'rice'.

2 Place a large frying pan over medium heat and heat the oil. Add the broccoli crumbs and lemon zest, and season with salt and pepper. Sauté for 3–5 minutes, or until the broccoli has softened.

3 Serve as a base for your favourite curry, stir-fry or anything else that is saucy and delicious.

SERVES 2–4 AS A SIDE

Cauliflower Mash

Beautiful
1 large head of cauliflower, chopped
1 clove garlic

Unstoppable
1 tablespoon coconut cream

Fearless
1 tablespoon ghee or vegan butter
1 cup nutritional yeast flakes
sea salt and pepper, to taste

1 Place the garlic, skin on, in the oven and roast for 10 minutes at 120°C. Place to one side to cool.

2 Steam the cauliflower for around 15 minutes, or until soft. Meanwhile, preheat a grill to medium-high.

3 Transfer the steamed cauliflower to a large bowl and, while it is still very hot, pop the garlic from its skin and add to the bowl. Add the ghee, ¾ of the nutritional yeast flakes, the coconut cream, salt and pepper. Mash the ingredients thoroughly.

4 Transfer to a serving bowl and top evenly with the remaining nutritional yeast flakes. Grill for 5 minutes, until browned.

Buf Girls' Tip

WE KNOW THAT INCLUDING AN INGREDIENT CALLED NUTRITIONAL YEAST IS A BIT 'WAY OUT', BUT WE PROMISE, YOU'LL TOTALLY LOVE IT! IT TASTES A LITTLE LIKE PARMESAN, IS GREAT FOR YOUR GUT HEALTH AND PACKED WITH VITAMINS.

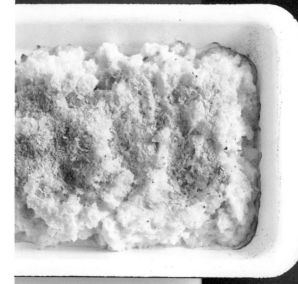

SERVES 2–4 AS A SIDE

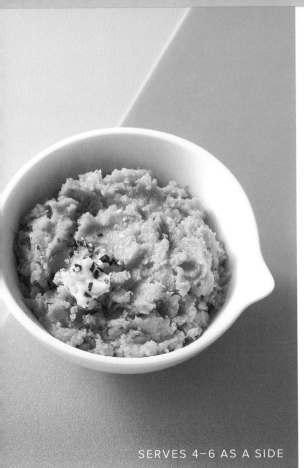

Sweet Potato Mash

Beautiful

2 large sweet potatoes

Unstoppable

1 heaped tablespoon ghee or vegan butter

Fearless

1 teaspoon chilli flakes

1 Peel the sweet potatoes, chop into cubes and boil until cooked through.
2 Remove from the heat, strain and place in a bowl containing the butter or ghee. Mash by hand, or purée with an electric mixer, until creamy and smooth. Stir chilli flakes through, and serve.

SERVES 4–6 AS A SIDE

Zapped and Zesty Greens
(for the time-poor BUF Girl)

Beautiful

1 cup chopped broccoli
1 tablespoon (or just 1 big squeeze) of lemon or lime juice

Unstoppable

drizzle of tahini (optional)

Fearless

sea salt and pepper, to taste

1 Place the broccoli in a microwave-safe bowl, add the juice and a little salt and pepper, then cover with a plate. Microwave on high for 90 seconds, then leave to rest for a minute or two.
2 Remove the plate, drain the liquid away and eat up! Those wanting a little extra yum factor can drizzle some tahini on top.

SERVES 1

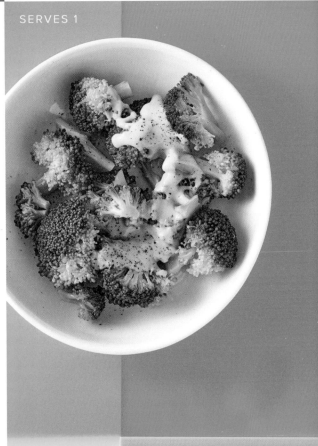

Pimped-up Nut Butter

Beautiful

2 tablespoons chia seeds
(optional)

Unstoppable

400 g roasted nuts of your choice
(e.g. almonds, cashews)

Fearless

1 tablespoon coconut oil
1 tablespoon cacao/cinnamon (optional)
1 teaspoon salt (optional)

1 Place the nuts in a blender and whiz on high until
they attain the consistency of butter.

2 Add the coconut oil, then add any flavour combos
you like: chia seeds, cacao/cinnamon and sea salt.
Blend until combined.

Cinnamon Roasted Pumpkin

Beautiful

half a medium-sized pumpkin (Japanese,
Kent or butternut)

Unstoppable

a drizzle of almond butter (optional)

Fearless

1 tablespoon olive oil
1 teaspoon cinnamon
sea salt, to taste

1 Preheat the oven to 180°C and line a tray with
baking paper.

2 Chop the pumpkin into small chunks and place
in a bowl. Add the olive oil and cinnamon and
massage with your hands to get even coverage.

3 Transfer the pumpkin to the tray and sprinkle
with a little salt. Bake for 45 minutes, or until the
pumpkin is cooked through and crispy on top.

4 Serve as a yummy side, adding an optional
teaspoon of almond butter if you're after
some protein.

SERVES 2–4

Spinach Bread

Beautiful

2 packets frozen spinach, thawed

Unstoppable

1 egg, lightly beaten (or vegan egg substitute)

Fearless

spices/herbs of your choice (e.g. garlic,
chilli, dill, nutmeg)
sea salt and pepper, to taste

1 Preheat the oven to 190°C and line a shallow baking
dish with baking paper.

2 Squeeze all the water out of the spinach and stir in the
egg. Add spices and herbs to taste, plus salt and pepper.

3 Press the mixture into the bottom of the prepared
dish and bake for 15–20 minutes.

4 Either eat immediately with poached eggs or baked
beans for breakfast (yum!), or cool and store individual
slices in the freezer to enjoy as snacks.

Kale Chips

Beautiful

½ bunch of kale, stalks removed and leaves
roughly chopped

Fearless

1 tablespoon olive oil
1 teaspoon paprika
2 tablespoons nutritional yeast flakes
1 teaspoon sea salt

1 Preheat the oven to 160°C and line a tray with
baking paper.

2 In a bowl, massage the chopped kale leaves
with olive oil. Add the paprika, nutritional yeast
flakes and sea salt and toss until the leaves are
thoroughly coated.

3 Tip the kale onto the baking tray and bake for
10 minutes, watching carefully to make sure they
don't burn. Allow to cook slightly, then eat away!

SERVES 2–3

Lettuce Wedges

Beautiful

¼ iceberg lettuce, chopped into chunks

Unstoppable

¼ cup natural yoghurt or coconut yoghurt
1 tablespoon pepitas

Fearless

1 teaspoon Dijon mustard
sea salt and pepper, to taste

In a bowl, mix together the yoghurt and Dijon mustard. Spread dollops of the yoghurt onto chunks of lettuce, season to taste and top with pepitas.

SERVES 1

Parsnip Chips

Beautiful

250 g parsnips

Unstoppable

2 tablespoons coconut oil

Fearless

sea salt and pepper, to taste

1 Preheat the oven to 200°C.
2 Wash the parsnips and cut into thin fries.
3 Melt the coconut oil in a roasting tin and toss in the parsnips, with salt and pepper. Roast for 15–20 minutes, or until golden brown, flipping them over halfway through the cooking time.

SERVES 2–3 AS A SIDE

Avocado and Chickpea Hummus

Beautiful

juice of ½ lemon
veggie sticks (e.g. carrot, capsicum, celery), to serve

Unstoppable

400 g can chickpeas, drained and rinsed
2 tablespoons tahini

Fearless

½ ripe avocado
1 tablespoon olive oil
1 teaspoon ground cumin
1 teaspoon sea salt
¼ cup water

1 Place all the ingredients in a blender and whiz until well combined. Serve with the veggie sticks.

SERVES 6

Rocket Pesto

Beautiful

2 cups rocket
1 handful of mint leaves

Unstoppable

½ cup almonds
¼ cup pistachios
¼ cup olive oil

Fearless

2 tablespoons nutritional yeast flakes
¼ cup water
1 teaspoon sea salt

1 Place all the ingredients in a blender and whiz until combined. You may need to add a touch more water if the pesto is too thick.

Celebratory Pina No-Colada

2 fresh dates, pitted
a few chunks of fresh or canned pineapple,
    chopped up
1 cup fresh coconut milk
pinch of cinnamon (or a little more if you like it spicy)
ice cubes

1 Pop all the ingredients in a blender, whiz until
   smooth and drink up!

SERVES 1

Mock Mojito

ice cubes
3 lime wedges
1 handful of mint leaves
sparkling water

1 Pop some ice cubes in a tall glass and squeeze lime
   wedges over it, then drop the wedges into
   your glass.
2 Squash the mint leaves between your hands
   to release the flavour, then drop these into the
   glass, too. Add sparkling water and enjoy!

SERVES 1

Perky Pear Martini

1 pear
half small fennel bulb
5 celery sticks
ice cubes

1 Roughly chop the pear, fennel and celery, feed
   through your juicer and pour the martini over ice.

SERVES 1

Buf Girls' Tip

YOU'LL NEED A JUICER AND A FANCY
GLASS FOR THIS ONE!

Mug of Triple C Goodness

pinch of cinnamon
1 heaped teaspoon carob powder
1 heaped teaspoon cacao powder
pinch of stevia
¼ cup milk of your choice
½–¾ cup boiling water

1 Combine the cinnamon, carob, cacao and stevia
   in a mug and stir vigorously with milk of your choice
   Add boiling water and you're done!

SERVES 1

Not-So-Bloody-Mary

4 celery sticks
2 tomatoes, peeled
1 teaspoon tamari
sea salt, to taste
filtered water

1 Juice three of the celery sticks.
2 Put the tomatoes and juiced celery into a blender, along with the tamari and salt to taste. Blend until smooth, adding filtered water as necessary, then pour into a tall glass and garnish with your final stick of celery.

SERVES 1

Protein-packed Super Smoothie

½ cup frozen mixed berries
1 handful of spinach leaves
½ cup milk of your choice
    (e.g. almond or coconut)
½ cup coconut water
1 serve of protein powder
1 tablespoon chia seeds

1 Place all the ingredients in a blender and whiz until smooth. We love ours with lots of ice!

SERVES 1

Buf Girls' Tip

YOU MIGHT ALSO LIKE TO ADD A SPOONFUL OF RAW CACAO FOR A LITTLE MORNING PEP-ME-UP, OR HALF A FROZEN BANANA FOR EXTRA ENERGY IF YOU'VE WORKED OUT IN THE MORNING.

Turmeric Chai

1 cup milk of your choice
1 teaspoon maple syrup or stevia
1 teaspoon coconut oil
1 teaspoon ground cinnamon
½ teaspoon ground turmeric
pinch of pepper

1 Combine all the ingredients in a saucepan and bring to a simmer. Simmer until warmed through.

SERVES 1

Vanilla Crush

½ frozen banana
1 Medjool date, pitted
1 cup milk of your choice
½ cup ice
1 teaspoon vanilla essence
1 teaspoon cinnamon
1 scoop coconut ice-cream (optional)

1 Place all the ingredients (except the coconut ice-cream) in a blender and whiz until smooth. Top with an optional scoop of ice-cream.

SERVES 1

Perfect 3 pm Fixes

APPLE WITH NUT BUTTER

Core and slice an apple and spread nut butter onto the slices. Top with a sprinkle of cinnamon or nutmeg, and enjoy. Apple is proven to wake you up more effectively than a shot of coffee, so go for it!

BANANA MINT DELIGHT

Place half a chopped frozen banana in a blender and add some cacao powder and mint leaves. If you like, you can also add a splash of coconut milk or almond milk. Blend on high for a few seconds and enjoy!

DANDELION MOCHA

In a mug, place 1 dandelion root tea bag, 1 teaspoon of raw cacao and a sweetener of your choice. Fill the mug ½–¾ with freshly boiled water, then top with almond milk.

DATE HEAVEN

Fill 2–3 fresh dates with ricotta or nut butter.

SALT AND VINEGAR ALMONDS

Pour 50 ml of apple cider vinegar and scatter 1 tablespoon of salt over 1½ cups of almonds, then roast in the oven at 180°C for 10–15 minutes.

SUPERFOOD TRAIL MIX

Mix together 20 goji berries, 10 almonds, 10 pistachios, 10 cashews and ¼ cup flaked coconut, then package up into snack-sized portions. Stash packets of this trail mix in your handbag or gym bag for a quick snack, or pair with some yoghurt and fruit for a filling snack. Feeling a little naughty? Add a square or two of chopped dark chocolate (we love 80–90% cacao).

VEGETABLE JUICE

Put kale, celery, carrot, ginger, lemon and ½ green apple through a juicer.

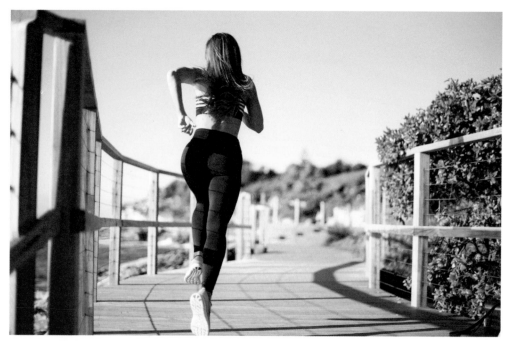

Dressings, Marinades & Sauces

FRENCH ONION DIP

1 tablespoon olive oil
2 cloves garlic, crushed
2 white onions, finely
    chopped
2 cups natural yoghurt or
    coconut yoghurt
1 tablespoon tamari
1 tablespoon balsamic vinegar

Heat a frying pan with olive oil
and cook the garlic and onion
for 5 minutes, or until the
onion is translucent. Allow to
cool completely. In a bowl, mix
together the cooked onion/
garlic, yoghurt, tamari and
vinegar. Stir well. Serve with
your choice of veggie sticks
or pita bread. This dip is also
perfect as a salad topper and
a dressing.

FRESH PESTO

4 cups fresh basil leaves,
    rinsed and dried
½ cup olive oil
⅓ cup pine nuts
⅓ cup cloves garlic
½ cup freshly grated
    Parmesan (or nutritional
    yeast flakes)
sea salt, to taste

Whiz all the ingredients
together in a food processor.
Transfer the pesto to a jar and
store in the fridge until ready
to use.

BALSAMIC VINAIGRETTE

2 tablespoons balsamic
    vinegar
1 tablespoon extra-virgin
    olive oil
1 tablespoon Dijon mustard
1 tablespoon dried thyme
salt and pepper, to taste

Mix all the ingredients
together in a jar. Shake
before use.

AVOCADO & CORIANDER DRESSING

½ soft avocado
1 tablespoon coconut yoghurt
1 tablespoon olive oil
1 tablespoon apple cider
    vinegar
8 sprigs of coriander
sea salt and pepper, to taste

Whiz all the ingredients
together in a food processor.
Transfer to a jar and shake
before use.

LEMONY HUMMUS DRESSING

1 tablespoon apple cider
    vinegar
juice of ½ lemon
2 tablespoons hummus

Mix all ingredients together
in a jar. Shake before use.

SIMPLE LEMON & OREGANO MARINADE

2 tablespoons extra-virgin
    olive oil or ghee
1 tablespoon finely chopped
    fresh oregano
3 cloves garlic, crushed
1 teaspoon onion powder
juice of ½ lemon

Mix all the ingredients together
in a bowl and marinate your
protein of choice in it.

TANGY CITRUS MUSTARD DRESSING

1 tablespoon olive oil
2 tablespoons fresh
    grapefruit juice
2 teaspoons apple cider
    vinegar
1 teaspoon Dijon mustard
1 teaspoon rice malt syrup
    (or raw honey or maple syrup)

Mix all the ingredients together
in a jar. Shake before use.

MUSTARD AVOCADO DRESSING

1 soft avocado
2 tablespoons Dijon mustard
1 tablespoon olive oil
2 tablespoons water

Whiz all the ingredients
together in a food processor.
Transfer to a jar and shake
before use.

Index

Resources to keep the fire burning

Now that you're starting to really get excited about living a Beautiful, Unstoppable and Fearless lifestyle, make sure you keep exploring, trying new things and learning everything you can. We've made a list of cool stuff you can read, watch, listen to and explore.

BOOKS

Libby loves
- *Gut* by Giulia Enders
- *In Defence of Food* by Michael Pollan
- *An Integrated Journey Back To Health and Happiness* by Dr Kate Wood

Cass loves
- *Live a Beautiful Life* by Jesinta Campbell
- *The Body Book* by Cameron Diaz
- *You Are Enough* by Cassie Mendoza-Jones

Leash loves
- *The Less Stress Lifestyle* by Carl Vernon
- *Sweet Poison* by David Gillespie
- *Woman Code* by Alisa Vitti

Sian loves
- *Rushing Woman's Syndrome* by Dr Libby Weaver
- *Supercharged Food* by Lee Holmes
- *Holistic Nutrition* by Kate Callaghan

PODCASTS

Libby loves
- 'TED Radio Hour' (TED Talks and TED Talks Health are great, too!)
- 'Eat, Move and Live Better' by Precision Nutrition

Cass loves
- 'Vibrant Happy Women'
- 'Dishing Up Nutrition'

Leash loves
- 'Wellness Women Radio'
- 'Let It Out with Katie Dalebout'

Sian loves
- 'Psychology of Eating'
- 'The Marie Forleo Podcast'

DOCUMENTARIES

Libby loves
- *Overfed and Undernourished*
- *Bolt*

Cass loves
- *That Sugar Film*
- *Miss Representation*

Leash loves
- *Happy*
- *Hungry For Change*

Sian loves
- *Embrace*
- *Marathon Challenge*